M|P|R

Medical Pocket Reference

DRUG-HERB INTERACTIONS

LIPPINCOTT WILLIAMS & WILKINS
A **Wolters Kluwer** Company
Philadelphia • Baltimore • New York • London
Buenos Aires • Hong Kong • Sydney • Tokyo

Staff

Publisher
Judy Schilling McCann, RN, MSN

Editorial Director
William J. Kelly

Senior Art Director
Arlene Putterman

Art Director
Elaine Kasmer

Clinical Manager
Eileen Cassin Gallen, RN, BSN

Senior Editor
Ann E. Houska

Drug Information Editor
Melissa M. Devlin, PharmD

Clinical Project Editor
Minh N. Luu, RN

Clinical Editor
Kimberly A. Zalewski, RN, MSN

Editor
Leanne Sullivan

Copy Editor
Leslie Dworkin

Electronic Production Services
Diane Paluba (manager), Joyce Rossi Biletz (senior desktop assistant), Donald G. Knauss (project manager)

Manufacturing
Patricia K. Dorshaw (manager), Beth Janae Orr (book production manager)

Editorial Assistants
Danielle J. Barsky, Carol A. Caputo, Arlene P. Claffee

Indexer
Deborah K. Tourtlotte

 For information, write Lippincott Williams & Wilkins, 1111 Bethlehem Pike, P.O. Box 908, Springhouse, PA 19477-0908.

Visit our Web site at eDrugInfo.com

ISBN 1-558255-220-7
MPRDHI—D N
05 04 03 02 10 9 8 7 6 5 4 3 2 1

Library of Congress Cataloging-in-Publication Data

Medical pocket reference : drug-herb interactions.
p.;cm.
Includes index.
1. Drug-herb interactions—Handbooks, manuals, etc.
[DNLM: 1. Pharmaceutical Preparations—Handbooks. 2. Plant Preparations—Handbooks. 3. Drug Interactions—Handbooks. 4. Phytotherapy—methods—Handbooks. QV 39 M4895 2003]
I. Title: Drug-herb interactions. II. Lippincott Williams & Wilkins.
RM302 .M435 2003
615'.7045—dc21 2002013635
ISBN 1-58255-220-7 (pbk.:alk. paper)

Contents

How to use this book

Medical Pocket Reference: Drug-Herb Interactions is designed to help you quickly find generic drugs and the herbs that interact with them. A list of all the abbreviations used in the book appears first. Then come the drug entries organized alphabetically by generic name. Next to each generic name you'll find common trade names, with Canadian names indicated by a diamond-shaped symbol (♦).

The first column in each drug entry lists the herbs that may interact with that particular drug. Herbs that may cause life-threatening interactions are shown in boldface type.

The second column in each drug entry lists the possible effects that may result from taking the herb and drug together.

The third column provides clinical tips for reducing, preventing, or managing the drug-herb interaction.

Appendices include normal laboratory test values and a listing of unsafe herbs.

The index contains herb and drug brand names.

Guide to abbreviations

AIDS	acquired immunodeficiency syndrome
am	morning
amt	amount
BP	blood pressure
chemo	chemotherapy
CrCl	creatinine clearance
d	day
div	divided
dl	deciliter
equiv	equivalent
eval	evaluation
exam	examination
g	gram
GI	gastrointestinal
gtt	drops
GU	genitourinary
h	hour
Hct	hematocrit
Hgb	hemoglobin
HIV	human immunodeficiency virus
hs	at bedtime
HSV	herpes simplex virus
HTN	hypertension
infect	infection
inhal	inhalant, inhalation
inhib	inhibitor
INR	international normalized ratio
IU	international unit
kg	kilogram
L	liter
LFT	liver function test
liq	liquid
m^2	square meter
MAO	monoamine oxidase
mEq	milliequivalent
mg	milligram
MI	myocardial infarction
min	minute
ml	milliliter
mo	month
NSAID	nonsteroidal anti-inflammatory drug
PO	by mouth
postop	postoperative
preop	preoperative
prep	preparation
prn	as needed
PT	prothrombin time
pt	patient
PTT	partial thromboplastin time
RF	renal failure
SSRI	selective serotonin reuptake inhibitor
supp	suppositories
suppl	supplement
syn	syndrome
TCA	tricyclic antidepressant
URI	upper respiratory tract infection
UTI	urinary tract infection
wk	week
wkly	weekly
wt	weight
yr	year

Herb	Possible effects	Clinical tips
abacavir sulfate • Ziagen		
bitter melon **fenugreek** **skullcap** **woundwort** **yerba maté**	May increase the risk of hepatotoxicity.	▪ Monitor pt for nausea, vomiting, jaundice, and elevated bilirubin level, which may indicate liver damage and hepatotoxicity.
boneset **butterbur** **chaparral** **coltsfoot** **comfrey**	Contains pyrrolizidine alkaloids, which may be hepatotoxic.	▪ Discourage use together. ▪ Monitor pt for signs and symptoms of liver damage, including abdominal pain, fever, malaise, jaundice, dark urine, clay-colored stools, and increased LFT values.
echinacea	May increase hepatotoxicity if used with drugs that raise liver enzyme levels. May exacerbate HIV by depressing CD+4 cells and increasing HIV replication.	▪ Discourage use in pt taking antiviral.
milk thistle	Liver membrane stabilization and antioxidant effects of this herb may protect against liver damage caused by various hepatotoxic drugs.	▪ Combination may be used for therapeutic advantage. ▪ Monitor LFT values.
abciximab • ReoPro		
angelica root anise arnica flower chamomile	May increase risk of bleeding because of coumarin or coumarin derivatives in herb. Herb may inhibit platelet activation factor, increasing bleeding times in susceptible pt.	▪ Monitor pt for signs and symptoms of increased bleeding, including bruising, petechiae, bleeding gums, epistaxis, prolonged bleeding after injury, melena, GI bleeding, hematuria, and hematemesis.

danshen devil's claw dong quai fenugreek garlic horse chestnut licorice papain parsley passion flower red clover reishi mushroom rue sweet clover		▪ Monitor results of hematologic studies and coagulation studies. ▪ Advise pt to consult health care provider before using herb.
bilberry bromelain clove ginkgo biloba onion turmeric	May increase risk of bleeding because of antiplatelet activity of herb.	▪ Monitor pt for signs and symptoms of increased bleeding, including bruising, petechiae, bleeding gums, epistaxis, prolonged bleeding after injury, melena, GI bleeding, hematuria, and hematemesis. ▪ Monitor results of hematologic studies and coagulation studies.
capsicum feverfew	May decrease platelet aggregation. May increase fibrolytic activity, which prolongs bleeding time.	▪ Monitor pt for signs and symptoms of increased bleeding, including bruising, petechiae, bleeding gums, epistaxis, prolonged bleeding after injury, melena, GI bleeding, hematuria, and hematemesis. ▪ Monitor results of hematologic studies and coagulation studies.

Herb	Possible effects	Clinical tips
abciximab *(continued)*		
coenzyme Q10 ginseng St. John's wort	May antagonize drug effects, lowering INR.	▪ Monitor PT and INR. ▪ Dosage adjustment may be needed.
echinacea	May increase bleeding time without elevating INR.	▪ Monitor pt for signs and symptoms of increased bleeding, including bruising, petechiae, bleeding gums, epistaxis, prolonged bleeding after injury, melena, GI bleeding, hematuria, and hematemesis. ▪ Monitor results of hematologic studies and coagulation studies.
ginger	Inhibits platelet aggregation by antagonizing thromboxane synthetase and enhancing prostacyclin. May prolong bleeding time.	▪ Monitor pt for signs and symptoms of increased bleeding, including bruising, petechiae, bleeding gums, epistaxis, prolonged bleeding after injury, melena, GI bleeding, hematuria, and hematemesis. ▪ Monitor results of hematologic studies and coagulation studies.
grapeseed	May increase drug effects and INR because of tocopherol content of herb.	▪ Monitor pt for signs and symptoms of increased bleeding, including bruising, petechiae, bleeding gums, epistaxis, prolonged bleeding after injury, melena, GI bleeding, hematuria, and hematemesis. ▪ Monitor results of hematologic and coagulation studies.
green tea nettle	May antagonize drug effects because of vitamin content in herb.	▪ Monitor pt for clinical effect. ▪ Monitor PT and INR. ▪ Dosage adjustment may be needed.

meadowsweet white willow	May increase risk of bleeding because of salicylates in herb.	▪ Monitor pt for signs and symptoms of increased bleeding, including bruising, petechiae, bleeding gums, epistaxis, prolonged bleeding after injury, melena, GI bleeding, hematuria, and hematemesis. ▪ Monitor results of hematologic and coagulation studies.

acarbose • Prandase ◆, Precose

aloe bilberry leaf bitter melon bladderwrack burdock dandelion fenugreek garlic ginseng	Use together may improve glucose control, requiring a reduction of antidiabetics. Herb may stimulate endogenous insulin release.	▪ Advise pt to consult health care provider before using herb. ▪ Monitor glucose level. ▪ Monitor pt for signs and symptoms of hypoglycemia, such as dizziness, diaphoresis, confusion, and tachycardia.
basil bay bee pollen burdock ginkgo biloba ginseng glucomannan horehound marshmallow myrrh sage	May affect glycemic control.	▪ Monitor glucose level. ▪ Monitor pt for signs and symptoms of hyperglycemia (fatigue, polyuria, polydipsia, wt loss, abdominal pain, altered mental status, tachycardia, hypotension, glucosuria, ketonuria). ▪ Monitor pt for signs and symptoms of hypoglycemia (dizziness, diaphoresis, confusion, tachycardia).

Herb	Possible effects	Clinical tips
acarbose *(continued)*		
bitter melon **fenugreek** **skullcap** **woundwort** **yerba maté**	May increase the risk of hepatotoxicity.	▪ Monitor pt for nausea, vomiting, jaundice, and elevated bilirubin level, which may indicate liver damage and hepatotoxicity.
boneset **butterbur** **chaparral** **coltsfoot** **comfrey**	Contains pyrrolizidine alkaloids, which may be hepatotoxic.	▪ Discourage use together. ▪ Monitor pt for signs and symptoms of liver damage, including abdominal pain, fever, malaise, jaundice, dark urine, clay-colored stools, and increased LFT values.
echinacea	May increase hepatotoxicity if used with drugs that raise liver enzyme levels.	▪ Discourage use in pt taking antiviral.
ma huang	May decrease hypoglycemic drug effect because of herb's hyperglycemic properties.	▪ Monitor glucose level. ▪ Monitor pt for signs and symptoms of hyperglycemia, such as fatigue, polyuria, polydipsia, wt loss, abdominal pain, altered mental status, tachycardia, hypotension, glucosuria, and ketonuria.
milk thistle	Liver membrane stabilization and antioxidant effects of herb may protect against liver damage caused by various hepatotoxic drugs. Herb may increase likelihood of loose stools, an adverse effect of acarbose.	▪ May be used for therapeutic advantage. ▪ Monitor LFT values.

senega root	May disrupt antidiabetic therapy. May cause hypoglycemia.	▪ Monitor glucose level closely. ▪ Dosage of antidiabetic may need to be adjusted.
yarrow	May cause hypoglycemia.	▪ Discourage use together because of herb's hypoglycemic properties.
acetaminophen • Feverall, Panadol, Tempra, Tylenol		
bitter melon **fenugreek** **skullcap** **woundwort** **yerba maté**	May increase the risk of hepatotoxicity.	▪ Monitor pt for nausea, vomiting, jaundice, and elevated bilirubin level, which may indicate liver damage and hepatotoxicity.
boneset **butterbur** **chaparral** **coltsfoot** **comfrey**	Contains pyrrolizidine alkaloids, which may be hepatotoxic.	▪ Discourage use together. ▪ Monitor pt for signs and symptoms of liver damage, including abdominal pain, fever, malaise, jaundice, dark urine, clay-colored stools, and increased LFT values.
coenzyme Q10 milk thistle	May protect liver against harmful effects of drug.	▪ May be used for therapeutic advantage.
echinacea	May increase hepatotoxicity if used with drugs that raise liver enzyme levels.	▪ Monitor LFT values. ▪ Monitor pt for signs and symptoms of hepatotoxicity.
watercress	May inhibit the oxidative metabolism of drug.	▪ Monitor pt for increased adverse effects, especially hepatotoxicity.

Herb	Possible effects	Clinical tips
acyclovir • Avirax ◆, Zovirax		
echinacea	May exacerbate HIV by depressing CD+4 cells and increasing HIV replication.	▪ Discourage use of herb in pt with HIV.
snakeroot	May increase risk of kidney problems because one component of snakeroot, aristolochic acid, has nephrotoxic properties.	▪ Discourage use of herb because of its toxic and carcinogenic potential.
allopurinol • Apo-Allopurinol ◆, Lopurin, Purinol ◆, Zyloprim		
bitter melon **fenugreek** **skullcap** **woundwort** **yerba maté**	May increase the risk of hepatotoxicity.	▪ Monitor pt for nausea, vomiting, jaundice, and elevated bilirubin level, which may indicate liver damage and hepatotoxicity.
boneset **butterbur** **chaparral** **coltsfoot** **comfrey**	Contains pyrrolizidine alkaloids, which may be hepatotoxic.	▪ Discourage use together. ▪ Monitor pt for signs and symptoms of liver damage, including abdominal pain, fever, malaise, jaundice, dark urine, clay-colored stools, and increased LFT values.
echinacea	May increase hepatotoxicity if used with drugs that raise liver enzyme levels.	▪ Advise pt to avoid use together if possible. ▪ Monitor LFT values.
kava valerian	May increase adverse CNS effects of drug.	▪ Monitor pt for increased sedation.
milk thistle	Liver membrane stabilization and antioxidant effects of herb may protect against liver	▪ May be used for therapeutic advantage. ▪ Monitor LFT values.

Herb	Interaction	Nursing considerations
	damage caused by various hepatotoxic drugs.	
snakeroot	May increase risk of kidney problems because one component of snakeroot, aristolochic acid, has nephrotoxic properties.	▪ Discourage use of herb because of its toxic and carcinogenic potential.
alprazolam • Alprazolam Intensol, Apo-Alpraz ◆, Novo-Alprazol ◆, Xanax		
ashwagandha capsicum catnip danshen goldenseal **kava** lady's slipper lemon balm linden melatonin nettle passion flower sassafras skullcap valerian root	May cause excessive physical depression, sedation, and impairment. Use of kava may cause coma.	▪ Signs and symptoms of toxicity are increased lethargy, disorientation, and daytime drowsiness. ▪ Advise pt to use together with caution and to avoid operating machinery or driving.
cola nut ephedra guarana yohimbe	May antagonize the anxiolytic effects of alprazolam.	▪ Signs and symptoms of use together include rapid heart rate, dizziness, and shortness of breath. ▪ Discourage use together.

Herb	Possible effects	Clinical tips
alprazolam *(continued)*		
St. John's wort	May decrease the muscle relaxant effects of the benzodiazepine.	▪ Monitor pt for loss of therapeutic effect. ▪ Advise pt to use together with caution.
amitriptyline hydrochloride • Apo-Amitriptyline ♦, Elavil, Endep, Levate ♦, Novotriptyn ♦		
angel's trumpet belladonna butterbur corkwood henbane jimsonweed	May increase anticholinergic effects.	▪ Monitor pt for increased adverse effects, including headache, dizziness, confusion, irritability, tachycardia, mydriasis, dry mouth, constipation, urinary retention, and hot, dry skin.
borage **fennel oil** **ginkgo** **sage** **St. John's wort** **wormwood**	May lower seizure threshold and increase risk of seizure, especially with higher than recommended doses of amitriptyline and in pt with seizure disorder.	▪ Discourage use together.
capsicum catnip goldenseal **kava** lady's slipper lemon balm melatonin nettle passion flower	May cause excessive physical depression, sedation, and impairment. Use of kava may cause coma.	▪ Monitor pt for signs and symptoms of increased CNS depression, including sedation, dizziness, ataxia, altered mental status, and respiratory depression.

sassafras skullcap valerian		
coenzyme Q10	May result in therapeutic failure of coenzyme Q10.	▪ Discourage use together. ▪ May deplete intracellular stores of coenzyme Q10.
evening primrose oil	May lower the seizure threshold and increase the risk for seizure activity.	▪ Discourage use together. ▪ Monitor pt for seizure activity.
SAMe **St. John's wort** **yohimbe**	May cause elevation of serotonin level.	▪ Discourage use together. ▪ Monitor pt for signs and symptoms of serotonin syn, including nausea, hypotension, HTN, excitation, mental status changes, hyperpyrexia, and coma.
yohimbe	May cause HTN in pt taking TCA.	▪ Discourage use together. ▪ Monitor BP.

amoxapine • Asendin

borage **fennel oil** **ginkgo** **St. John's wort** **wormwood**	May further lower the seizure threshold.	▪ Discourage use together. ▪ Monitor pt for seizure activity.
capsicum catnip goldenseal **kava** lady's slipper lemon balm	May cause excessive physical depression, sedation, and impairment. Use of kava may cause coma.	▪ Monitor pt for signs and symptoms of increased CNS depression, including sedation, dizziness, ataxia, altered mental status, and respiratory depression.

Herb	Possible effects	Clinical tips
amoxapine *(continued)*		
melatonin nettle passion flower sassafras skullcap valerian	May cause excessive physical depression, sedation, and impairment.	▪ Monitor pt for signs and symptoms of increased CNS depression, including sedation, dizziness, ataxia, altered mental status, and respiratory depression.
evening primrose oil	May lower the seizure threshold and increase the risk of seizure activity.	▪ Discourage use together. ▪ Monitor pt for seizure activity.
SAMe **St. John's wort** **yohimbe**	May elevate serotonin level.	▪ Discourage use together. ▪ Monitor pt for signs and symptoms of serotonin syn, including nausea, hypotension, HTN, excitation, mental status changes, hyperpyrexia, and coma.
amprenavir • Agenerase		
echinacea	May exacerbate HIV infection or AIDS by depressing CD+4 cells and increasing HIV replication.	▪ Discourage use together.
garlic	May cause severe GI toxicity when used together with ritonavir. May reduce effectiveness of some drugs used for HIV.	▪ Discourage use together.
St. John's wort	Reduces indinavir level by more than 50%. May have similar effects with other protease inhibitors.	▪ Discourage use together.

aspirin • ASA, Ascriptin, Bufferin, Ecotrin		
angelica root anise arnica flower chamomile danshen devil's claw dong quai fenugreek garlic horse chestnut licorice papain parsley passion flower red clover reishi mushroom rue sweet clover	May increase risk of bleeding because of coumarin or coumarin derivatives in herb. Herb may inhibit platelet activation factor. May increase bleeding time in susceptible pt.	▪ Monitor pt for signs and symptoms of increased bleeding, including bruising, petechiae, bleeding gums, epistaxis, prolonged bleeding after injury, melena, GI bleeding, hematuria, and hematemesis. ▪ Monitor results of hematologic studies and coagulation studies. ▪ Advise pt to consult health care provider before using herb.
bilberry bromelain clove feverfew ginkgo biloba horse chestnut	May increase risk of bleeding because of antiplatelet activity of herb.	▪ Discourage use together. ▪ Tell pt to report unusual bruising or bleeding. ▪ Monitor PT and INR.

Herb	Possible effects	Clinical tips
aspirin *(continued)*		
onion prickly ash turmeric	May increase risk of bleeding because of antiplatelet activity of herb.	▪ Discourage use together. ▪ Tell pt to report unusual bruising or bleeding. ▪ Monitor PT and INR.
capsicum feverfew	May decrease platelet aggregation. May increase fibrolytic activity, which prolongs bleeding time.	▪ Monitor pt for signs and symptoms of increased bleeding, including bruising, petechiae, bleeding gums, epistaxis, prolonged bleeding after injury, melena, GI bleeding, hematuria, and hematemesis. ▪ Monitor results of hematologic studies and coagulation studies.
echinacea	May increase bleeding time without elevating INR.	▪ Monitor pt for signs and symptoms of increased bleeding, including bruising, petechiae, bleeding gums, epistaxis, prolonged bleeding after injury, melena, GI bleeding, hematuria, and hematemesis.
ginger	Inhibits platelet aggregation by antagonizing thromboxane synthetase and enhancing prostacyclin, prolonging bleeding time.	▪ Monitor pt for signs and symptoms of increased bleeding, including bruising, petechiae, bleeding gums, epistaxis, prolonged bleeding after injury, melena, GI bleeding, hematuria, and hematemesis. ▪ Monitor results of hematologic studies and coagulation studies.
grapeseed	May increase drug effects and INR because of tocopherol content of herb.	▪ Monitor pt for signs and symptoms of increased bleeding, including bruising, petechiae, bleeding gums, epistaxis, prolonged bleeding after injury, melena, GI bleeding, hematuria, and hematemesis.

		▪ Monitor results of hematologic studies and coagulation studies.
meadowsweet white willow	May increase risk of bleeding because of salicylates in herb. May increase other adverse effects of aspirin.	▪ Monitor pt for signs and symptoms of increased bleeding, including bruising, petechiae, bleeding gums, epistaxis, prolonged bleeding after injury, melena, GI bleeding, hematuria, and hematemesis. ▪ Monitor pt for signs and symptoms of aspirin toxicity, including lethargy, tinnitus, GI discomfort, oliguria, acute RF, hyperthermia, tachypnea, acid-base imbalances, dehydration, pulmonary edema, and tachycardia.
atenolol • Apo-Atenol ◆, Tenormin		
black cohosh	May increase peripheral vasodilation, resulting in hypotension.	▪ Monitor BP closely. ▪ Dosage adjustment may be needed.
ephedra	May increase BP because of unopposed sympathetic stimulation.	▪ Monitor pt for changes in BP and heart rate, arrhythmias, and shortness of breath.
ginger	May antagonize antihypertensive effect of drug.	▪ Monitor BP.
goldenseal	May interfere with drug's action because the alkaloids of the herb have hypertensive properties.	▪ Advise pt of this effect. ▪ Monitor BP.
licorice	May increase sodium, chloride, and H_2O retention, resulting in BP increase.	▪ Monitor BP.
mistletoe	May interfere with therapeutic drug effects. Viscotoxins in herb may produce reflex	▪ Monitor pt's vital signs and ECG for arrhythmias.

(continued)

Herb	Possible effects	Clinical tips
atenolol *(continued)*		
mistletoe *(continued)*	bradycardia and have negative inotropic effects on cardiac muscle.	
yohimbe bark	May cause a decrease in drug effect because of hypertensive effects of herb.	▪ Advise pt of this effect. ▪ Monitor BP closely.
atorvastatin • Lipitor		
bitter melon **fenugreek** **skullcap** **woundwort** **yerba maté**	May increase the risk of hepatotoxicity.	▪ Monitor pt for nausea, vomiting, jaundice, and elevated bilirubin level, which may indicate liver damage and hepatotoxicity.
boneset **butterbur** **chaparral** **coltsfoot** **comfrey**	Contains pyrrolizidine alkaloids, which may be hepatotoxic.	▪ Discourage use together. ▪ Monitor pt for signs and symptoms of liver damage, including abdominal pain, fever, malaise, jaundice, dark urine, clay-colored stools, and increased LFT values.
coenzyme Q10	May result in therapeutic failure of coenzyme Q10.	▪ Discourage use together. ▪ Drug may deplete intracellular stores of coenzyme Q10.
coltsfoot **kava**	May increase the risk of hepatotoxicity.	▪ Monitor LFT values closely. ▪ Advise pt to avoid using together.
echinacea	May increase hepatotoxicity if used with drugs that raise liver enzyme levels.	▪ Monitor LFT values.

Herb	Effect	Nursing considerations
garlic	May have additive lipid-lowering properties.	▪ May be used together for therapeutic advantage.
milk thistle	Liver membrane stabilization and antioxidant effects of herb may protect against liver damage caused by various hepatotoxic drugs.	▪ May be used together for therapeutic advantage. ▪ Monitor LFT values.
pectin	May decrease the effectiveness of HMG-CoA reductase inhibitors.	▪ Discourage use together. ▪ Monitor pt for clinical response.
red yeast rice	Contains components similar to those of statin drugs, increasing the risk of adverse events or toxicity.	▪ Advise pt to avoid use together if possible. ▪ Monitor pt for signs and symptoms of adverse effects such as myopathy and rhabdomyolysis (increased creatinine kinase level, muscle aches, weakness) or increased LFT values.
St. John's wort	May decrease blood level of drugs in the statin family, leading to failure of drug therapy.	▪ Monitor pt for clinical response. ▪ Discourage use together.
benazepril • Lotensin		
birch dandelion goldenrod uva-ursi	May antagonize antihypertensive effects of benazepril.	▪ Advise pt to use together with caution. ▪ Monitor BP.
black cohosh	May increase peripheral vasodilation, resulting in hypotension.	▪ Monitor BP closely. ▪ Dosage adjustment may be needed.
capsaicin	Increases risk of cough.	▪ Discourage use together.

Herb	Possible effects	Clinical tips
benazepril *(continued)*		
ephedra	May antagonize antihypertensive effects of benazepril. May cause HTN and tachycardia.	▪ Discourage use together. ▪ Advise pt to report dizziness, rapid heart rate, headache, and incoordination to health care provider immediately.
ginger	May antagonize antihypertensive effect.	▪ Monitor BP closely. ▪ Dosage adjustment may be needed.
glucosamine	May antagonize antihypertensive effect. May cause hyperkalemia. Depending on the specific product, glucosamine may contain high concentrations of sodium or potassium.	▪ Monitor pt's BP or potassium level, depending on glucosamine prep. ▪ Advise pt with HTN, HF, or renal dysfunction to select a product low in sodium or potassium.
goldenseal	May interfere with drug's antihypertensive effects because the herb's alkaloids have hypertensive properties.	▪ Monitor pt for clinical effect. ▪ Monitor BP.
laminaria L-arginine	May increase risk of hyperkalemia. May increase potassium level.	▪ Monitor potassium level and renal function. ▪ Discourage use together.
licorice	May increase sodium, chloride, and H_2O retention, resulting in BP increase.	▪ Monitor BP.
white willow	May antagonize drug's antihypertensive effects. May inhibit production of prostaglandins, including vasodilator and antithrombotic prostaglandins.	▪ Monitor BP. ▪ Advise pt to use together with caution.

yohimbe bark	May cause a decrease in drug effect because of hypertensive effects of herb.	▪ Monitor BP closely. ▪ Dosage adjustment may be needed.
bepridil hydrochloride • Vascor		
aloe **buckthorn** **cascara sagrada** **Chinese rhubarb** **frangula** **guarana** **licorice** **ma huang** **senna**	May change cardiac rhythm and increase the potential for arrhythmias because herb causes hypokalemia.	▪ Monitor potassium levels. ▪ Monitor pt for signs and symptoms of hypokalemia, including muscle weakness, fatigue, nausea, vomiting, constipation, respiratory depression, and arrhythmias.
cat's claw chicory	May increase antianginal effect.	▪ Advise pt to consult health care provider before taking herb.
ginger	May increase calcium uptake by the myocardium, leading to altered drug effects.	▪ Monitor pt for therapeutic effect. ▪ Discourage use together.
bumetanide • Bumex		
agrimony bitter orange coriander dong quai fennel khella	Loop diuretics may increase photosensitivity, adding to the risk of sunburn or skin rash.	▪ Advise pt to wear sunscreen or protective clothing during sun exposure if he uses herb while taking a loop diuretic.

Herb	Possible effects	Clinical tips
bumetanide *(continued)*		
lovage motherwort Queen Anne's lace rosemary (topical) St. John's wort	Loop diuretics may increase photosensitivity, adding to the risk of sunburn or skin rash.	▪ Advise pt to wear sunscreen or protective clothing during sun exposure if he uses herb while taking a loop diuretic.
aloe	Loop diuretics cause additive potassium-wasting effect.	▪ Monitor potassium level. ▪ Monitor pt for signs and symptoms of hypokalemia, including muscle weakness, fatigue, nausea, vomiting, constipation, respiratory depression, and arrhythmias.
artichoke dandelion goldenseal gossypol	May potentiate effect of diuretic. May increase risk of hypokalemia.	▪ Monitor potassium level. ▪ Discourage use during diuretic therapy.
dandelion uva-ursi	May decrease effect of diuretic because of the sodium-sparing effect of herb.	▪ Monitor pt for therapeutic effect of drug. ▪ Discourage use during diuretic therapy.
ginseng	Decreases effect of diuretic.	▪ Monitor pt for therapeutic effect of drug. ▪ Discourage use during diuretic therapy.
licorice	May cause unexpectedly rapid potassium loss. However, deglycyrrhizinated licorice shouldn't affect potassium levels.	▪ Monitor potassium level. ▪ Monitor pt for signs and symptoms of hypokalemia, including muscle weakness, fatigue, nausea, vomiting, constipation, respiratory depression, and arrhythmias.

bupropion • Wellbutrin, Wellbutrin SR, Zyban

Herb	Effect	Nursing considerations
borage **fennel oil** **ginkgo** **St. John's wort** **wormwood**	May lower the seizure threshold.	▪ Discourage use together. ▪ Monitor pt for seizure activity..
capsicum catnip goldenseal **kava** lady's slipper lemon balm melatonin nettle passion flower sassafras skullcap valerian	May cause excessive physical depression, sedation, and impairment. Use of kava may cause coma.	▪ Monitor pt for signs and symptoms of increased CNS depression, including sedation, dizziness, ataxia, and altered mental status.
evening primrose oil	May lower the seizure threshold and increase the risk of seizure activity.	▪ Discourage use together. ▪ Monitor pt for seizure activity.
St. John's wort	May have MAO inhibitor properties.	▪ Discourage use together. ▪ MAO inhibitors may alter the seizure threshold in pt also taking bupropion.

Herb	Possible effects	Clinical tips
buspirone • BuSpar		
capsicum catnip goldenseal **kava** lady's slipper lemon balm melatonin nettle passion flower sassafras skullcap valerian	May cause excessive physical depression, sedation, and impairment. Use of kava may cause coma.	▪ Monitor pt for signs and symptoms of increased CNS depression, including sedation, dizziness, ataxia, and altered mental status.
St. John's wort	May have MAO inhibitor properties.	▪ Discourage use together. ▪ Monitor BP. MAO inhibitors may increase BP in pt also taking buspirone.
captopril • Capoten, Novo-Captoril ♦		
black catechu	May increase herb's hypotensive effect.	▪ Monitor BP. ▪ Dosage adjustment may be needed.
black cohosh	May increase peripheral vasodilation, resulting in hypotension.	▪ Monitor BP closely. ▪ Dosage adjustment may be needed.
capsaicin	May increase risk of cough.	▪ Discourage use to avoid increased risk of cough.
ginger	May antagonize drug's antihypertensive effect.	▪ Monitor BP closely. ▪ Dosage adjustment may be needed.

goldenseal	May interfere with drug's action because alkaloids of herb have hypertensive properties.	▪ Monitor pt for clinical effect. ▪ Monitor BP.
licorice	May cause sodium retention and increase BP, interfering with the therapeutic effects of ACE inhibitors.	▪ Advise pt of this interaction. ▪ Monitor BP.
yohimbe bark	May cause a decrease in drug effect because of hypertensive effects of herb.	▪ Monitor BP closely. ▪ Dosage adjustment may be needed.
carbamazepine • Apo-Carbamazepine ♦, Atretol, Carbatrol, Epitol, Novo-Carbamaz ♦, Tegretol, Tegretol CR ♦, Tegretol-XR		
borage **fennel oil** **ginkgo** **St. John's wort** **wormwood**	May decrease effectiveness of anticonvulsants.	▪ Discourage use together.
evening primrose oil	May lower the seizure threshold.	▪ Discourage use together. ▪ Monitor pt for loss of therapeutic effect of drug.
hyssop	May counteract the antiseizure effects of anticonvulsants.	▪ Discourage use together. ▪ Monitor pt for loss of therapeutic effect of drug.
nettle	May increase sedative adverse effects. May increase risk of seizures.	▪ Discourage use together.
plantain	May inhibit absorption of drug in the GI tract, decreasing serum concentration.	▪ Monitor pt for lack or loss of therapeutic effect. ▪ Advise pt not to take herb during drug therapy.
sage	May induce seizures.	▪ Advise pt to use together cautiously.

Herb	Possible effects	Clinical tips
carvedilol • Coreg		
black cohosh	May increase peripheral vasodilation, resulting in hypotension.	▪ Monitor BP closely. ▪ Dosage adjustment may be needed.
ephedra	May increase BP because of unopposed sympathetic stimulation.	▪ Monitor pt for changes in BP and heart rate, arrhythmias, and shortness of breath.
ginger	May antagonize antihypertensive effect.	▪ Monitor BP.
goldenseal	May interfere with drug's action because the alkaloids of herb have hypertensive properties.	▪ Advise pt of this effect. ▪ Monitor BP.
licorice	May increase sodium, chloride, and H_20 retention, resulting in BP increase.	▪ Monitor BP.
saw palmetto	May have an additive alpha adrenergic blocking effect when combined with alpha blockers.	▪ Monitor vital signs and ECG for adverse effects.
yohimbe bark	May decrease drug's effectiveness because of hypertensive effects of herb.	▪ Advise pt of this effect. ▪ Monitor BP closely.
celecoxib • Celebrex		
angelica root anise arnica flower bilberry	May increase risk of bleeding because of coumarin or coumarin derivatives in herb or because of antiplatelet activity of herb.	▪ Monitor pt for signs and symptoms of increased bleeding, including bruising, petechiae, bleeding gums, epistaxis, prolonged bleeding after injury, melena, GI bleeding, hematuria, and hematemesis.

bromelain capsicum chamomile clove danshen devil's claw dong quai echinacea fenugreek feverfew garlic ginger ginkgo biloba horse chestnut licorice onion papain parsley passion flower red clover reishi mushroom rue sweet clover turmeric	May inhibit platelet activation factor, increasing bleeding times in susceptible people.	▪ Monitor results of hematologic studies and coagulation studies. ▪ Advise pt to consult health care provider before using herb.
bitter melon **fenugreek** **skullcap**	May increase risk of hepatotoxicity.	▪ Monitor pt for nausea, vomiting, jaundice, and elevated bilirubin level, which may indicate liver damage and hepatotoxicity.

Interacting herbs in **bold type** indicate life-threatening interactions. ◆ Canadian

Herb	Possible effects	Clinical tips
celecoxib *(continued)*		
woundwort **yerba maté**	May increase risk of hepatotoxicity.	▪ Monitor pt for nausea, vomiting, jaundice, and elevated bilirubin level, which may indicate liver damage and hepatotoxicity.
bitter orange coriander dong quai fennel khella lovage motherwort Queen Anne's lace rosemary (topical) St. John's wort	May increase photosensitivity.	▪ Advise pt to avoid unprotected exposure to sunlight.
boneset **butterbur** **chaparral** **coltsfoot** **comfrey**	Contains pyrrolizidine alkaloids, which may be hepatotoxic.	▪ Discourage use together. ▪ Monitor pt for signs and symptoms of liver damage, including abdominal pain, fever, malaise, jaundice, dark urine, clay-colored stools, and increased LFT values.
capsicum	May stimulate GI secretions to help protect against NSAID-induced GI irritation.	▪ Combination may be used for therapeutic advantage.
Coffea arabica cola	May increase adverse GI effects.	▪ Advise pt of increased risk of adverse GI effects.

Herb	Effect	Nursing considerations
gossypol uva-ursi		
echinacea	May increase hepatotoxicity if used with drugs that raise liver enzyme levels.	▪ Advise pt of this adverse effect. ▪ Monitor LFT values.
meadowsweet white willow	May increase risk of bleeding because of salicylates in herb.	▪ Discourage use together.
milk thistle	Liver membrane stabilization and antioxidant effects of herb may protect against liver damage caused by various hepatotoxic drugs.	▪ May be used for therapeutic advantage. ▪ Monitor LFT values.
wild yam	May decrease the anti-inflammatory effect of drug.	▪ Monitor pt for clinical effect.
chlorpromazine • Chlorpromanyl-20 ♦, Chlorpromanyl-40 ♦, Largactil ♦, Thorazine		
kava	May cause tremors, muscle spasms, or abnormal movements. May decrease effectiveness of drug therapy.	▪ Warn pt not to use together. ▪ Any musculoskeletal or nervous system abnormalities should be promptly reported to health care provider.
cidofovir • Vistide		
bitter melon **fenugreek** **skullcap** **woundwort** **yerba maté**	May increase risk of hepatotoxicity.	▪ Monitor pt for nausea, vomiting, jaundice, and elevated bilirubin level, which may indicate liver damage and hepatotoxicity.

Herb	Possible effects	Clinical tips
cidofovir *(continued)*		
boneset **butterbur** **chaparral** **coltsfoot** **comfrey**	Contains pyrrolizidine alkaloids, which may be hepatotoxic.	▪ Monitor pt for signs and symptoms of liver damage, including abdominal pain, fever, malaise, jaundice, dark urine, clay-colored stools, and increased LFT values.
echinacea	May increase hepatotoxicity if used with drugs that raise liver enzyme levels. May exacerbate HIV by depressing CD+4 cells and increasing HIV replication.	▪ Discourage use in pt taking antiviral.
milk thistle	Liver membrane stabilization and antioxidant effects of herb may protect against liver damage caused by various hepatotoxic drugs.	▪ May be used for therapeutic advantage. ▪ Monitor LFT values.
snakeroot	May increase risk of kidney problems because one component of snakeroot, aristolochic acid, has nephrotoxic properties.	▪ Discourage use of herb because of its toxic and carcinogenic potential.
cimetidine • Tagamet, Tagamet HB		
blessed thistle bogbean capsicum ginger goldenseal mustard	May decrease effectiveness because of increased acid secretion caused by herb.	▪ Discourage use together.

yerba maté	May decrease clearance of herb's methylxanthines, causing toxicity.	▪ Discourage use together. ▪ Monitor pt for increased adverse effects, such as increased CNS stimulation or hepatotoxicity.

ciprofloxacin • Cipro, Cipro I.V.

agrimony bitter orange coriander dong quai fennel khella lovage motherwort Queen Anne's lace rosemary (topical) St. John's wort	May increase photosensitivity, adding to the risk of sunburn or skin rash.	▪ Advise pt to wear sunscreen or protective clothing during sun exposure.
borage **fennel oil** **ginkgo** **St. John's wort** **wormwood**	May reduce the seizure threshold and increase risk of seizures.	▪ Discourage use together. ▪ Monitor pt for seizure activity.
echinacea	May increase hepatotoxicity if used with drugs that raise liver enzyme levels.	▪ Advise pt of this adverse effect. ▪ Monitor LFT values.

Herb	Possible effects	Clinical tips
ciprofloxacin *(continued)*		
evening primrose oil	May lower the seizure threshold and increase the risk of seizure activity.	▪ Discourage use together. ▪ Monitor pt for seizure activity.
fennel	May reduce blood levels of drug, possibly impairing drug's effectiveness. May interfere similarly with other fluoroquinolone antibiotics.	▪ Advise pt to avoid, if possible, use of herb with this drug and other fluoroquinolone antibiotics. Otherwise, advise pt to separate use by 2 h to reduce the potential for an interaction. Emphasize that this may not eliminate the risk of interaction.
yerba maté	May decrease clearance of herb's methylxanthines, causing toxicity.	▪ Discourage use together. Monitor pt for increased adverse effects, such as increased CNS stimulation or hepatotoxicity.
citalopram • Celexa		
ginkgo	May reduce the sexual adverse effects of SSRIs in both men and women.	▪ Advise pt of this effect.
5-HTP **SAMe**	May cause serotonin syn.	▪ Discourage use together. ▪ Monitor pt for signs and symptoms, including nausea, hypotension, HTN, excitation, mental status changes, hyperpyrexia, and coma.
St. John's wort	May cause serotonin syn.	▪ Discourage use together. ▪ Advise pt switching from an SSRI to herb to wait a few wk for drug to leave his system before using herb. The exact time required depends on the SSRI being used. ▪ Advise pt to consult health care provider before using herb.
yohimbe	May cause serotonin syn.	▪ Discourage use together.

		▪ Monitor pt for nausea, hypotension, HTN, excitation, mental status changes, hyperpyrexia, and coma.
clonazepam • Klonopin, Rivotril ◆		
capsicum catnip goldenseal **kava** lady's slipper lemon balm melatonin nettle passion flower sassafras skullcap valerian	May cause excessive physical depression, sedation, and impairment. Use of kava may cause coma.	▪ Discourage use together. ▪ Monitor pt for signs and symptoms of increased CNS depression, including sedation, dizziness, ataxia, altered mental status, and respiratory depression.
linden	May increase side effects of benzodiazepine because herb has similar components.	▪ Advise pt not to take excessive amt of herb.
colchicine		
autumn crocus	May increase the risk of adverse reactions and toxicity because colchicine is the main active component in autumn crocus.	▪ Discourage use together. ▪ Monitor pt for signs and symptoms of toxicity, including nausea, vomiting, abdominal pain, and diarrhea. Diarrhea may be severe and bloody from hemorrhagic gastroenteritis. Burning sensations in the throat, stomach, and skin also may occur.
echinacea	May increase hepatotoxicity if used with drugs that raise liver enzyme levels.	▪ Advise pt of this adverse effect. ▪ Monitor LFT values.

Herb	Possible effects	Clinical tips
cyclobenzaprine • Flexeril		
butterbur corkwood henbane jimsonweed	May increase anticholinergic adverse effects.	▪ Monitor pt for increased adverse effects, including headache, drowsiness, dizziness, confusion, irritability, tachycardia, mydriasis, dry mouth, constipation, urinary retention, and hot, dry skin.
capsicum catnip goldenseal **kava** lady's slipper lemon balm melatonin nettle passion flower sassafras skullcap valerian	May cause excessive physical depression, sedation, and impairment. Use of kava may cause coma.	▪ Monitor pt for signs and symptoms of increased CNS depression, including sedation, dizziness, ataxia, altered mental status, and respiratory depression.
St. John's wort	Herb may have MAO inhibitor properties, which may cause hyperpyretic crisis, seizures, and even death when taken with drug.	▪ Discourage use together.
cyclosporine (cyclosporin A) • Neoral, Sandimmune		
alfalfa astragalus echinacea	May interfere with immunosuppressive effect of drug.	▪ Advise pt of this possible effect. ▪ Discourage use together. ▪ Watch for loss of therapeutic effect of drug.

European mistletoe licorice morinda		
bitter melon **fenugreek** **skullcap** **woundwort** **yerba maté**	May increase the risk of hepatotoxicity.	▪ Monitor pt for nausea, vomiting, jaundice, and elevated bilirubin level, which may indicate liver damage and hepatotoxicity.
boneset **butterbur** **chaparral** **coltsfoot** **comfrey**	Contains pyrrolizidine alkaloids, which may be hepatotoxic.	▪ Monitor pt for signs and symptoms of liver damage, including abdominal pain, fever, malaise, jaundice, dark urine, clay-colored stools, and increased LFT values.
echinacea	May increase hepatotoxicity if used with drugs that raise liver enzyme levels.	▪ Advise pt of this adverse effect. ▪ Monitor LFT values.
larch	May interfere with immunosuppressive actions of drug because herb contains arabinogalactans, polysaccharides that have immune-boosting properties.	▪ Advise pt of this possible effect. ▪ Discourage use together.
melatonin	May interfere with immunosuppression by improving immune function.	▪ Discourage use together because it could defeat the purpose of the immunosuppressive therapy.
milk thistle	Liver membrane stabilization and antioxidant effects of herb may protect against liver	▪ Combination may be used for therapeutic advantage. ▪ Monitor LFT values.

(continued)

Herb	Possible effects	Clinical tips
cyclosporine (cyclosporin A) *(continued)*		
milk thistle *(continued)*	damage caused by various hepatotoxic drugs.	
pill-bearing spurge	May inhibit CYP3A enzymes affecting drug metabolism.	▪ Use together cautiously. ▪ Monitor pt for adverse effects.
snakeroot	May increase risk of kidney problems because one component of snakeroot, aristolochic acid, has nephrotoxic properties.	▪ Discourage use of herb because of its toxic and carcinogenic potential.
St. John's wort	May decrease cyclosporine levels because of metabolic induction of the CYP 3A4 isoenzyme. May lead to organ rejection or require increased cyclosporine dosage.	▪ Advise pt to avoid using together. ▪ Monitor cyclosporine levels. If pt stops taking herb during therapy, monitor cyclosporine levels for possible dosage reduction. ▪ Monitor pt for loss of therapeutic effectiveness.
desipramine hydrochloride • Norpramin, Pertofrane ♦		
borage **fennel oil** **ginkgo** **wormwood**	May reduce the seizure threshold.	▪ Discourage use together. ▪ Monitor pt for seizure activity.
butterbur corkwood henbane jimsonweed	May increase anticholinergic effects.	▪ Monitor pt for increased adverse effects, including headache, dizziness, confusion, irritability, tachycardia, mydriasis, dry mouth, constipation, urinary retention, and hot, dry skin.
capsicum	May cause excessive physical depression,	▪ Monitor pt for signs and symptoms of increased CNS depres-

catnip goldenseal **kava** lady's slipper lemon balm melatonin nettle passion flower sassafras skullcap valerian	sedation, and impairment. Use of kava may cause coma.	sion, including sedation, dizziness, ataxia, altered mental status, and respiratory depression.
evening primrose oil	May lower the seizure threshold and increase the risk of seizure activity.	▪ Discourage use together. ▪ Monitor pt for seizure activity.
sage	May induce seizures.	▪ Discourage use together.
SAMe **St. John's wort** **yohimbe**	May cause elevation of serotonin level.	▪ Discourage use together. ▪ Monitor pt for signs and symptoms of serotonin syn, including nausea, hypotension, HTN, excitation, mental status changes, hyperpyrexia, and coma.
yohimbe	May cause HTN in pt taking TCA.	▪ Discourage use together. ▪ Monitor BP.

dexamethasone • Decadron, Deronil ♦, Dexasone ♦, Dexone, Hexadrol, Mymethasone

alfalfa astragalus echinacea	May interfere with immunosuppressive effect of drug.	▪ Advise pt of this possible effect. ▪ Discourage use together. ▪ Watch for loss of therapeutic effect of drug.

Herb	Possible effects	Clinical tips
dexamethasone *(continued)*		
European mistletoe morinda	May interfere with immunosuppressive effect of drug.	▪ Advise pt of this possible effect. ▪ Discourage use together. ▪ Watch for loss of therapeutic effect of drug.
licorice	May interfere with immunosuppressive effect of drug. May increase dexamethasone plasma levels and potentiate drug effects.	▪ Monitor pt for loss of therapeutic effect. ▪ Monitor pt for signs and symptoms of corticosteroid toxicity.
melatonin	May interfere with immunosuppression by improving immune function.	▪ Discourage use together as this may defeat the purpose of the immunosuppressive therapy.
dextromethorphan hydrobromide • Balminil DM, Benylin DM, Broncho-Grippol-DM, Buckley's DM, Children's Hold, Delsym, Hold DM, Koffex DM ◆, Pertussin CS, Pertussin ES, Robitussin Pediatric, St. Joseph Cough Suppressant, Sucrets Cough Control, Trocal, Vicks 44 Cough Relief		
St. John's wort	May have MAO inhibitor properties.	▪ Discourage use together. ▪ Risk of hypotension, coma, hyperpyrexia, and death when drug used with MAO inhibitors.
diazepam • Apo-Diazepam ◆, Diastat, Diazemuls ◆, Diazepam Intensol, Novo-Dipam ◆, PMS-Diazepam ◆, Valium, Vivol ◆		
capsicum catnip goldenseal **kava** lady's slipper lemon balm melatonin	May cause excessive physical depression, sedation, and impairment. Use of kava may cause coma.	▪ Discourage use together. ▪ Monitor pt for signs and symptoms of increased CNS depression, including sedation, dizziness, ataxia, altered mental status, and respiratory depression.

nettle passion flower sassafras skullcap valerian		
echinacea	May increase hepatotoxicity if used with drugs that raise liver enzyme levels. Some herbal tinctures contain a high concentration of alcohol (up to 90%).	▪ Advise pt of this adverse effect. ▪ Monitor LFT values. ▪ Pt should check the tincture's alcohol content before engaging in potentially hazardous activities that require mental alertness and coordination.
ephedra	Herb directly stimulates the sympathetic nervous system and may decrease the antianxiety or sedative properties of the drug.	▪ Monitor pt for decreased effectiveness of diazepam. ▪ Discourage use together.
linden	May increase side effects of benzodiazepine because herb contains similar components.	▪ Advise pt not to take excessive amt of herb.
digoxin • Digoxin, Lanoxicaps, Lanoxin, Novo-Digoxin ◆		
aloe **black root** **blue flag** **buckthorn** **butternut bark** **cascara bark** **castor oil**	May contribute to potassium loss, which increases the potential for drug toxicity resulting from hypokalemia.	▪ Monitor potassium and drug levels. Drug has a narrow therapeutic index. ▪ Monitor pt for signs and symptoms of drug toxicity, including fatigue, asthenia, dizziness, arrhythmias, visual disturbances, nausea, vomiting, and diarrhea.

Herb	Possible effects	Clinical tips
digoxin *(continued)*		
Chinese rhubarb **frangula** **gamboge** **guarana** **jalap root** **licorice** **podophyllum** **senna leaves and pods** **wild cucumber** **yellow dock root**	May contribute to potassium loss, which increases the potential for drug toxicity resulting from hypokalemia.	▪ Monitor potassium and drug levels. Drug has a narrow therapeutic index. ▪ Monitor pt for signs and symptoms of drug toxicity, including fatigue, asthenia, dizziness, arrhythmias, visual disturbances, nausea, vomiting, and diarrhea.
betel palm fumitory goldenseal lily-of-the-valley motherwort rue shepherd's purse	May enhance cardiac effects.	▪ Discourage use together. ▪ Monitor pt for increased cardiac effects, including severe bradycardia, hypotension, and arrhythmias. ▪ Advise pt to consult health care provider before using herb.
eleuthero-coccus senticosus **hawthorn**	May increase the risk of drug toxicity because of cardiac glycoside content in herb.	▪ Discourage use together. ▪ Monitor drug level.

Herb	Effect	Nursing considerations
Siberian ginseng **uzara** **yellow foxglove**		
ephedra	May cause CV instability.	▪ Discourage use of herb.
fenugreek flaxseed	May alter the absorption of drug because of the fibrous content and binding properties of herb.	▪ Advise pt to separate administration times by > 2 h to prevent decreased absorption. ▪ Monitor pt for decreased effects of drug.
ginger	Herb contains cardiotonic components (gingerols, volatile oils, and other compounds) that have positive inotropic effects. May interfere pharmacodynamically with drug.	▪ Monitor heart rate. ▪ Watch for increased effects of drug.
ginseng	May falsely elevate digoxin level.	▪ Advise pt of this effect. ▪ Monitor serum level.
kyushin	May interfere with determination of drug level.	▪ Discourage use together to obtain reliable drug level.
ma huang	Increases risk of arrhythmias.	▪ Discourage use together.
plantain	May cause decreased drug absorption, resulting in decreased therapeutic effects.	▪ Advise pt to separate administration times. ▪ Monitor pt for therapeutic effect.
rauwolfia	May cause severe bradycardia when used in combination with drug.	▪ Discourage use together. ▪ Monitor vital signs and ECG closely.

Herb	Possible effects	Clinical tips
digoxin *(continued)*		
squill	Potentiates the positive inotropic and negative chronotropic effects of drug.	▪ Monitor pt for increased effects. ▪ Dosage adjustment may be needed.
St. John's wort	May cause decreased drug level, resulting in decreased therapeutic effects.	▪ Advise pt of this interaction. ▪ Monitor drug level.
diltiazem • Apo-Diltiaz ◆, Cardizem, Cardizem CD, Cardizem SR, Dilacor XR, Tiazac		
aloe **buckthorn** **cascara sagrada** **Chinese rhubarb** **frangula** **guarana** **licorice** **ma huang** **senna**	May cause a change in cardiac rhythm and increase the potential for arrhythmias because hypokalemia is associated with use of herb.	▪ Monitor potassium level. ▪ Monitor pt for signs and symptoms of hypokalemia, including muscle weakness, fatigue, nausea, vomiting, constipation, respiratory depression, and arrhythmias.
black cohosh	Increases peripheral vasodilation, resulting in hypotension.	▪ Monitor BP closely. ▪ Dosage adjustment may be needed.
cat's claw chicory	May increase antianginal effect of drug.	▪ Advise pt to consult health care provider before using herb.
ginger	May increase calcium uptake by the myocardium, leading to altered drug effects.	▪ Monitor pt for therapeutic effect. ▪ Discourage use together.

goldenseal	May interfere with drug's action because the alkaloids of herb have hypertensive properties.	▪ Monitor pt for clinical effect. ▪ Monitor BP.
licorice	May increase sodium, chloride, and H_2O retention, resulting in BP increase.	▪ Monitor BP.
yohimbe bark	May cause a decrease in drug effect because of hypertensive effects of herb.	▪ Monitor BP closely. ▪ Dosage adjustment may be needed.
diphenhydramine hydrochloride • Allerdryl ◆, Banophen, Beldin, Belix, Benadryl, Benylin, Bydramine Cough, Compoz, Diphen Cough, Diphenadryl, Diphenhist, Hydramine, Nervine Nighttime Sleep-Aid, Sleep-eze 3, Sominex, Tusstat, Twilite Caplets		
butterbur corkwood henbane jimsonweed	May increase anticholinergic adverse effects.	▪ Monitor pt for increased adverse effects, including headache, drowsiness, dizziness, confusion, irritability, tachycardia, mydriasis, dry mouth, constipation, urinary retention, and hot, dry skin.
capsicum catnip goldenseal **kava** lady's slipper lemon balm melatonin nettle passion flower sassafras skullcap valerian	May cause excessive physical depression, sedation, and impairment. Use of kava may cause coma.	▪ Monitor pt for signs and symptoms of increased CNS depression, including sedation, drowsiness, dizziness, ataxia, altered mental status, and respiratory depression.

Herb	Possible effects	Clinical tips
diphenhydramine hydrochloride *(continued)*		
St. John's wort	May have MAO inhibitor properties; MAO inhibitor use increases anticholinergic effects.	▪ Discourage use together.
docetaxel • Taxotere		
boneset **butterbur** **chaparral** **coltsfoot** **comfrey**	Contains pyrrolizidine alkaloids, which may be hepatotoxic.	▪ Monitor pt for signs and symptoms of liver damage, including abdominal pain, fever, malaise, jaundice, dark urine, clay-colored stools, and increased LFT values.
echinacea	May increase hepatotoxicity if used with drugs that raise liver enzyme levels.	▪ Advise pt of this adverse effect. ▪ Monitor LFT values.
ginger	May decrease nausea caused by chemo.	▪ May be used for this therapeutic effect.
milk thistle	Liver membrane stabilization and antioxidant effects of herb may protect against liver damage caused by various hepatotoxic drugs.	▪ Combination may be used for therapeutic advantage. ▪ Monitor LFT values.
St. John's wort	May decrease the effectiveness of drug, requiring a dosage adjustment.	▪ Discourage use together. ▪ Health care provider should select an appropriate antidepressant for pt.
yew	May potentiate myelosuppression and interactions with other chemo drugs.	▪ Warn pt about this possible interaction.

dofetilide • Tikosyn

Herb	Effect	Action
aloe **buckthorn** **cascara sagrada** **Chinese rhubarb** **frangula** **guarana** **licorice** **ma huang** **senna**	May cause a change in cardiac rhythm and increase the potential for arrhythmias because hypokalemia is associated with use of herb.	▪ Monitor pt for signs and symptoms of hypokalemia, including muscle weakness, fatigue, nausea, vomiting, constipation, respiratory depression, and arrhythmias.
boneset **butterbur** **chaparral** **coltsfoot** **comfrey**	Contains pyrrolizidine alkaloids, which may be hepatotoxic.	▪ Monitor pt for signs and symptoms of liver damage, including abdominal pain, fever, malaise, jaundice, dark urine, clay-colored stools, and increased LFT values.
echinacea	May increase hepatotoxicity if used with drugs that raise liver enzyme levels.	▪ Advise pt of this adverse effect. ▪ Monitor LFT values.
milk thistle	Liver membrane stabilization and antioxidant effects of herb may protect against liver damage caused by various hepatotoxic drugs.	▪ Combination may be used for therapeutic advantage. ▪ Monitor LFT values.

Herb	Possible effects	Clinical tips
doxepin hydrochloride • Adapin, Novo-Doxepin ◆, Sinequan, Triadapin ◆		
belladonna butterbur corkwood henbane jimsonweed	Increases anticholinergic effects.	▪ Monitor pt for increased adverse effects, including headache, dizziness, confusion, irritability, tachycardia, mydriasis, dry mouth, constipation, urinary retention, and hot, dry skin.
borage **fennel oil** **ginkgo** **St. John's wort** **wormwood**	May lower the seizure threshold.	▪ Discourage use together. ▪ Monitor pt for seizure activity.
capsicum catnip goldenseal **kava** lady's slipper lemon balm melatonin nettle passion flower sassafras skullcap valerian	May cause excessive physical depression, sedation, and impairment. Use of kava may cause coma.	▪ Monitor pt for signs and symptoms of increased CNS depression, including sedation, dizziness, ataxia, altered mental status, and respiratory depression.
evening primrose oil	May lower the seizure threshold and increase the risk of seizure activity.	▪ Discourage use together. ▪ Monitor pt for seizure activity.

Herb	Interaction	Nursing considerations
SAMe **St. John's wort** **yohimbe**	May cause elevation of serotonin level.	▪ Discourage use together. ▪ Monitor pt for signs and symptoms of serotonin syn, including nausea, hypotension, HTN, excitation, mental status changes, hyperpyrexia, and coma.
doxycycline • Apo-Doxy ◆, Doryx, Doxy Caps, Doxycin ◆, Novo-Doxylin ◆, Vibramycin, Vibra-Tabs		
agrimony bitter orange coriander dong quai fennel khella lovage motherwort Queen Anne's lace rosemary (topical) St. John's wort	May increase photosensitivity, adding to the risk of sunburn or skin rash.	▪ Advise pt to wear a sunscreen or protective clothing during sun exposure.
echinacea	May increase hepatotoxicity if used with drugs that raise liver enzyme levels. May exacerbate tuberculosis.	▪ Discourage use together.
Siberian ginseng	May enhance the effects of some antibiotics.	▪ May be used for therapeutic advantage.
enalapril • Vasotec		
agrimony bitter orange	May increase photosensitivity, adding to the risk of sunburn or skin rash.	▪ Advise pt to wear a sunscreen or protective clothing during sun exposure.

Herb	Possible effects	Clinical tips
enalapril *(continued)*		
coriander dong quai fennel khella lovage motherwort Queen Anne's lace rosemary (topical) St. John's wort	May increase photosensitivity, adding to the risk of sunburn or skin rash.	▪ Advise pt to wear a sunscreen or protective clothing during sun exposure.
black cohosh	May increase peripheral vasodilation, resulting in hypotension.	▪ Monitor BP closely. ▪ Dosage adjustment may be needed.
capsaicin	May increase risk of cough.	▪ Pt may want to avoid this combination to avoid increased risk of cough.
ginger	May antagonize antihypertensive effect of drug.	▪ Monitor BP closely. ▪ Dosage adjustment may be needed.
goldenseal	May interfere with drug's action because the alkaloids of herb have hypertensive properties.	▪ Monitor pt for clinical effect. ▪ Monitor BP.
licorice	May cause sodium retention and increase BP, interfering with the therapeutic effects of ACE inhibitors.	▪ Advise pt of this interaction. ▪ Monitor BP.

Herb	Interaction	Nursing considerations
yohimbe bark	May cause a decrease in drug effect because of hypertensive effects of herb.	▪ Monitor BP closely. ▪ Dosage adjustment may be needed.
enoxaparin sodium • Lovenox		
angelica root anise arnica flower chamomile danshen devil's claw dong quai fenugreek garlic horse chestnut licorice papain parsley passion flower red clover reishi mushroom rue sweet clover	May increase risk of bleeding because of coumarin or coumarin derivatives in herb. May inhibit platelet activation factor, increasing bleeding times in susceptible people.	▪ Monitor pt for signs and symptoms of increased bleeding, including bruising, petechiae, bleeding gums, epistaxis, prolonged bleeding after injury, melena, GI bleeding, hematuria, and hematemesis. ▪ Monitor results of hematologic studies and coagulation studies. ▪ Advise pt to consult health care provider before using herb.
bilberry bromelain clove ginkgo biloba	May increase risk of bleeding because of antiplatelet activity of herb.	▪ Monitor pt for signs and symptoms of increased bleeding, including bruising, petechiae, bleeding gums, epistaxis, prolonged bleeding after injury, melena, GI bleeding, hematuria, and hematemesis.

(continued)

Herb	Possible effects	Clinical tips
enoxaparin sodium *(continued)*		
onion turmeric		▪ Monitor results of hematologic studies and coagulation studies.
capsicum feverfew	Decreases platelet aggregation and increases fibrolytic activity, prolonging bleeding time.	▪ Monitor pt for signs and symptoms of increased bleeding, including bruising, petechiae, bleeding gums, epistaxis, prolonged bleeding after injury, melena, GI bleeding, hematuria, and hematemesis. ▪ Monitor results of hematologic studies and coagulation studies.
echinacea	May increase bleeding time without elevating INR.	▪ Monitor pt for signs and symptoms of increased bleeding, including bruising, petechiae, bleeding gums, epistaxis, prolonged bleeding after injury, melena, GI bleeding, hematuria, and hematemesis.
ginger	Inhibits platelet aggregation by antagonizing thromboxane synthetase and enhancing prostacyclin, prolonging bleeding time.	▪ Monitor pt for signs and symptoms of increased bleeding, including bruising, petechiae, bleeding gums, epistaxis, prolonged bleeding after injury, melena, GI bleeding, hematuria, and hematemesis. ▪ Monitor results of hematologic studies and coagulation studies.
goldenseal	May counteract the anticoagulant effect of enoxaparin sodium.	▪ Monitor results of hematologic studies and coagulation studies. ▪ Monitor pt for clinical effect.
grapeseed	Increases drug effects and INR because of tocopherol content of herb.	▪ Monitor pt for signs and symptoms of increased bleeding, including bruising, petechiae, bleeding gums, epistaxis, pro-

etodolac • Lodine, Lodine XL

Herb	Effect	Nursing considerations
agrimony bitter orange coriander dong quai fennel khella lovage motherwort Queen Anne's lace rosemary (topical) St. John's wort	May increase photosensitivity, adding to risk of sunburn or skin rash.	▪ Advise pt to wear a sunscreen or protective clothing during sun exposure.
angelica root anise arnica flower bilberry bromelain capsicum chamomile clove danshen devil's claw dong quai echinacea fenugreek	May increase risk of bleeding because of coumarin or coumarin derivatives in herb or because of antiplatelet activity of herb. May inhibit platelet activation factor, increasing bleeding times in susceptible individuals.	▪ Monitor pt for signs and symptoms of increased bleeding, including bruising, petechiae, bleeding gums, epistaxis, prolonged bleeding after injury, melena, GI bleeding, hematuria, and hematemesis. ▪ Monitor results of hematologic studies and coagulation studies. ▪ Advise pt to consult health care provider before using herb.

Herb	Possible effects	Clinical tips
etodolac *(continued)*		
feverfew garlic ginger ginkgo biloba horse chestnut licorice onion papain parsley passion flower red clover reishi mushroom rue sweet clover turmeric	May increase risk of bleeding because of coumarin or coumarin derivatives in herb or because of antiplatelet activity of herb. May inhibit platelet activation factor, increasing bleeding times in susceptible individuals.	▪ Monitor pt for signs and symptoms of increased bleeding, including bruising, petechiae, bleeding gums, epistaxis, prolonged bleeding after injury, melena, GI bleeding, hematuria, and hematemesis. ▪ Monitor results of hematologic studies and coagulation studies. ▪ Advise pt to consult health care provider before using herb.
balsam of Peru **fumitory** **gossypol** **juniper** **monascus** **oak bark** **rue** **soapwort**	Increases the risk of renal toxicity.	▪ Discourage use together. ▪ Monitor renal function tests.

thunder god vine **wild ginger** **wintergreen** **yohimbe**		
boneset **butterbur** **chaparral** **coltsfoot** **comfrey**	Contains pyrrolizidine alkaloids, which may be hepatotoxic.	▪ Discourage use together. ▪ Monitor pt for signs and symptoms of liver damage, including abdominal pain, fever, malaise, jaundice, dark urine, clay-colored stools, and increased LFT values.
capsicum	Stimulates GI secretions to help protect against NSAID-induced GI irritation.	▪ May be used for therapeutic advantage.
Coffea arabica cola gossypol uva-ursi	May increase hepatotoxicity if used with drugs that raise liver enzyme levels.	▪ Advise pt of this adverse effect. ▪ Monitor LFT values.
echinacea	May increase adverse GI effects.	▪ Advise pt of increased risk of adverse GI effects.
meadowsweet white willow	May increase risk of bleeding because of salicylates in herb.	▪ Monitor pt for signs and symptoms of increased bleeding, including bruising, petechiae, bleeding gums, epistaxis, prolonged bleeding after injury, melena, GI bleeding, hematuria, and hematemesis. ▪ Monitor results of hematologic studies and coagulation studies.
milk thistle	Liver membrane stabilization and antioxidant effects of herb may protect against liver	▪ Combination may be used for therapeutic advantage. ▪ Monitor LFT values.

(continued)

Interacting herbs in **bold type** indicate life-threatening interactions. ◆ Canadian

Herb	Possible effects	Clinical tips
etodolac *(continued)*		
milk thistle *(continued)*	damage caused by various hepatotoxic drugs.	
snakeroot	May increase risk of kidney problems because one component of snakeroot, aristolochic acid, has nephrotoxic properties.	▪ Discourage use of herb because of its toxic and carcinogenic potential.
wild yam	May decrease the anti-inflammatory effect of drug.	▪ Monitor pt for clinical effects.
famciclovir • Famvir		
echinacea	May exacerbate HIV by depressing CD+4 cells and increasing HIV replication.	▪ Advise pt with HIV to avoid herb if taking antiviral.
famotidine • Mylanta-AR, Pepcid, Pepcid AC, Pepcid RPD		
blessed thistle bogbean capsicum ginger goldenseal mustard	May decrease effectiveness because of increased acid secretion by herb.	▪ Advise pt of this effect. ▪ Monitor pt for clinical effect.
echinacea	May increase hepatotoxicity if used with drugs that raise liver enzyme levels.	▪ Advise pt of this adverse effect. ▪ Monitor LFT values.
milk thistle	Liver membrane stabilization and antioxidant effects of herb may protect against liver	▪ Combination may be used for therapeutic advantage. ▪ Monitor LFT values.

	damage caused by various hepatotoxic drugs.	
felodipine • Plendil, Renedil ♦		
black cohosh	May increase peripheral vasodilation, resulting in hypotension.	▪ Monitor BP closely. ▪ Dosage adjustment may be needed.
ginger	May increase calcium uptake by the myocardium, leading to altered drug effects.	▪ Monitor BP closely. ▪ Dosage adjustment may be needed.
goldenseal	May interfere with drug's action because herb has hypertensive properties.	▪ Monitor BP closely. ▪ Monitor pt for clinical effect.
licorice	May increase sodium, chloride, and H_20 retention, resulting in BP increase.	▪ Monitor BP closely.
yohimbe bark	May cause a decrease in drug effect because of hypertensive effects of herb.	▪ Monitor BP closely. ▪ Dosage adjustment may be needed.
ferrous sulfate • Apo-Ferrous Sulfate ♦, Feosol, Fer-gen-sol, Fer-In-Sol Syrup, Fer-Iron Drops, Fero-Grad, Mol-Iron		
black cohosh chamomile feverfew gossypol hawthorn nettle plantain saw palmetto St. John's wort valerian	May decrease iron absorption because herb contains tannin; tannin-iron complex may form.	▪ Monitor pt for adequate response to iron therapy.

Herb	Possible effects	Clinical tips
ferrous sulfate *(continued)*		
oregano	May reduce iron absorption.	▪ Advise pt to separate administration times by > 2 h when given with iron suppl or iron-containing foods.
rose hip	May increase iron absorption.	▪ Advise pt to separate administration times.
fexofenadine hydrochloride • Allegra		
kava valerian	May increase sedative effects of drug.	▪ Monitor pt for increased fatigue or drowsiness.
flecainide acetate • Tambocor		
aloe **buckthorn** **cascara sagrada** **Chinese rhubarb** **frangula** **guarana** **licorice** **ma huang** **senna**	May cause change in cardiac rhythm and increase potential for arrhythmias because herb causes hypokalemia.	▪ Monitor potassium level. ▪ Monitor pt for signs and symptoms of hypokalemia, such as muscle weakness, fatigue, nausea, vomiting, constipation, respiratory depression, and arrhythmias.
fluconazole • Diflucan		
boneset **butterbur** **chaparral**	Contains pyrrolizidine alkaloids, which may be hepatotoxic.	▪ Discourage use together. ▪ Monitor pt for signs and symptoms of liver damage, including abdominal pain, fever, malaise, jaundice, dark urine, clay-

Herb	Effect	Nursing considerations
coltsfoot **comfrey**		colored stools, and increased LFT values.
echinacea	May increase hepatotoxicity if used with drugs that raise liver enzyme levels.	▪ Advise pt of this adverse effect. ▪ Monitor LFT values.
milk thistle	Liver membrane stabilization and antioxidant effects of herb may protect against liver damage caused by various hepatotoxic drugs.	▪ Combination may be used for therapeutic advantage. ▪ Monitor LFT values.
fluoxetine • Prozac, Sarafem		
capsicum catnip goldenseal **kava** lady's slipper lemon balm melatonin nettle passion flower sassafras skullcap valerian	May cause excessive physical depression, sedation, and impairment. Use of kava may cause coma.	▪ Monitor pt for signs and symptoms of increased CNS depression, including sedation, drowsiness, dizziness, ataxia, altered mental status, and respiratory depression.
5-HTP **SAMe** **yohimbe**	May reduce the sexual adverse effects of SSRIs in both men and women.	▪ Advise pt of this effect.

Herb	Possible effects	Clinical tips
fluoxetine *(continued)*		
ginkgo	May cause serotonin syn if herb is combined with drugs that raise serotonin level, such as SSRIs.	▪ Discourage use together. ▪ Monitor pt for nausea, hypotension, HTN, excitation, mental status changes, hyperpyrexia, and coma.
melatonin	Drug may decrease endogenous levels of melatonin, which may result in disrupted sleep cycles.	▪ May improve sleep quality.
St. John's wort	May cause serotonin syn if herb is combined with drugs that raise serotonin level, such as SSRIs.	▪ Discourage use together. ▪ Pt switching from an SSRI to herb must wait a few wk for drug to leave his system before using herb. The exact time required depends on the SSRI being used. ▪ Advise pt to consult health care provider before using herb.
fluphenazine decanoate • Modecate ◆, Modecate Concentrate ◆, Prolixin Decanoate		
agrimony bitter orange coriander dong quai fennel khella lovage motherwort Queen Anne's lace rosemary (topical)	May increase photosensitivity, adding to the risk of sunburn or skin rash.	▪ Advise pt to wear a sunscreen or protective clothing during sun exposure.

betel nut	May increase cholinergic activity because of arecoline. May produce muscle rigidity, tremor, stiffness, akathisia, or bradykinesia.	▪ Advise pt to report use to health care provider. ▪ Musculoskeletal or nervous system side effects should be reported immediately.
boneset **butterbur** **chaparral** **coltsfoot** **comfrey**	Contains pyrrolizidine alkaloids, which may be hepatotoxic.	▪ Monitor pt for signs and symptoms of liver damage, including abdominal pain, fever, malaise, jaundice, dark urine, clay-colored stools, and increased LFT values.
borage **fennel oil** **ginkgo** **St. John's wort** **wormwood**	May lower the seizure threshold.	▪ Discourage use together. ▪ Monitor pt for seizure activity.
butterbur corkwood henbane jimsonweed	Increases anticholinergic effects.	▪ Advise pt of this interaction. ▪ Monitor pt for increased adverse effects, including headache, dizziness, confusion, irritability, tachycardia, mydriasis, dry mouth, constipation, urinary retention, and hot, dry skin.
capsicum catnip goldenseal **kava** lady's slipper lemon balm	May cause excessive physical depression, sedation, and impairment. Use of kava may cause coma.	▪ Monitor pt for signs and symptoms of increased CNS adverse effects, including sedation, dizziness, drowsiness, ataxia, and altered mental status.

Herb	Possible effects	Clinical tips
fluphenazine decanoate *(continued)*		
melatonin nettle passion flower sassafras skullcap valerian	May cause excessive physical depression, sedation, and impairment.	▪ Monitor pt for signs and symptoms of increased CNS adverse effects, including sedation, dizziness, drowsiness, ataxia, and altered mental status.
echinacea	May increase hepatotoxicity if used with drugs that raise liver enzyme levels.	▪ Advise pt of this adverse effect. ▪ Monitor LFT values.
evening primrose oil	May lower the seizure threshold and increase the risk of seizure activity.	▪ Discourage use together. ▪ Monitor pt for seizure activity.
ginseng	May increase CNS stimulant activity.	▪ Discourage use with antipsychotics.
hyssop **sage**	May counteract the antiseizure effects of anticonvulsants.	▪ Discourage use together. ▪ Monitor pt for loss of therapeutic effect of drug.
kava	May increase the risk or severity of dystonic reactions.	▪ Discourage use together.
milk thistle	Silymarin (contained in herb) in combination with phenothiazines causes a decrease in lipid peroxidation.	▪ May be used for therapeutic advantage to lessen hepatotoxicity.
yohimbe	Phenothiazine meds may increase the risk of toxicity.	▪ Discourage use together. ▪ Monitor pt for increased nervousness, headache, dizziness, mania or psychoses, tachycardia, hypotension or HTN, GI complaints, and RF.

flurazepam hydrochloride • Apo-Flurazepam ◆, Dalmane, Novo-Flupam ◆

Herb	Interaction	Action
capsicum catnip goldenseal **kava** lady's slipper lemon balm melatonin nettle passion flower sassafras skullcap valerian	May cause excessive physical depression, sedation, and impairment. Use of kava may cause coma.	▪ Advise pt to use together cautiously. ▪ Pt should discontinue valerian use before starting sedative therapy. ▪ Warn pt of overdrowsiness. Advise caution when operating a car or heavy machinery.
linden	May increase side effects of benzodiazepine because herb contains similar components.	▪ Advise pt not to use excessive amt of herb.

fluvastatin • Lescol

Herb	Interaction	Action
boneset **butterbur** **chaparral** **coltsfoot** **comfrey**	Contains pyrrolizidine alkaloids, which may be hepatotoxic.	▪ Discourage use together. ▪ Monitor pt for signs and symptoms of liver damage, including abdominal pain, fever, malaise, jaundice, dark urine, clay-colored stools, and increased LFT values.
echinacea	May increase hepatotoxicity if used with drugs that raise liver enzyme levels.	▪ Monitor LFT values.
garlic	May have additive lipid-lowering properties.	▪ May be used for therapeutic advantage.

Herb	Possible effects	Clinical tips
fluvastatin *(continued)*		
milk thistle	Liver membrane stabilization and antioxidant effects of herb may protect against liver damage caused by various hepatotoxic drugs.	▪ Combination may be used for therapeutic advantage. ▪ Monitor LFT values.
pectin	May decrease the effectiveness of HMG-CoA reductase inhibitors.	▪ Discourage use together. ▪ Monitor pt for clinical response.
red yeast rice	Contains similar components to those of statin drugs, increasing the risk of adverse events or toxicity.	▪ Discourage use together if possible. If must be used together, monitor pt for signs and symptoms of increased adverse effects, such as myopathy and rhabdomyolysis (increased creatinine kinase level, muscle aches, weakness) or increased LFT values.
St. John's wort	May decrease blood levels of various drugs in the statin family.	▪ Monitor pt for clinical response.
foscarnet • Foscavir		
boneset **butterbur** **chaparral** **coltsfoot** **comfrey**	Contains pyrrolizidine alkaloids, which may be hepatotoxic.	▪ Monitor pt for signs and symptoms of liver damage, including abdominal pain, fever, malaise, jaundice, dark urine, clay-colored stools, and increased LFT values.
echinacea	May increase hepatotoxicity if used with drugs that raise liver enzyme levels. May exacerbate HIV by depressing CD+4 cells	▪ Discourage use in pt taking antiviral.

	and increasing HIV replication.	
milk thistle	Liver membrane stabilization and antioxidant effects of herb may protect against liver damage caused by various hepatotoxic drugs.	▪ Combination may be used for therapeutic advantage. ▪ Monitor LFT values
snakeroot	May increase risk of kidney problems because one component of snakeroot, aristolochic acid, has nephrotoxic properties.	▪ Discourage use of herb because of its toxic and carcinogenic potential.
fosinopril • Monopril		
agrimony bitter orange coriander dong quai fennel khella lovage motherwort Queen Anne's lace rosemary (topical) St. John's wort	May increase photosensitivity, adding to the risk of sunburn or skin rash.	▪ Advise pt to wear a sunscreen or protective clothing during sun exposure.
black catechu	May increase hypotensive effect of herb.	▪ Monitor BP. ▪ Dosage adjustment may be needed.

Herb	Possible effects	Clinical tips
fosinopril *(continued)*		
black cohosh	May increase peripheral vasodilation, resulting in hypotension.	▪ Monitor BP closely. ▪ Dosage adjustment may be needed.
capsaicin	May increase risk of cough.	▪ Pt may want to avoid this combination to avoid increased risk of cough.
ginger	May antagonize antihypertensive effect.	▪ Monitor BP closely. ▪ Dosage adjustment may be needed.
goldenseal	May interfere with drug's action because the alkaloids of herb have hypertensive properties.	▪ Monitor pt for clinical effect. ▪ Monitor BP.
licorice	May cause sodium retention and increase BP, interfering with the therapeutic effects of ACE inhibitors.	▪ Advise pt of this interaction. ▪ Monitor BP.
yohimbe bark	May cause a decrease in drug effect because of hypertensive effects of herb.	▪ Monitor BP closely. ▪ Dosage adjustment may be needed.
fosphenytoin sodium • Cerebyx		
borage **fennel oil** **ginkgo** **St. John's wort** **wormwood**	May decrease effectiveness of anticonvulsants.	▪ Advise pt with seizure disorder to avoid herb.

Herb	Effect	Nursing considerations
echinacea	May increase hepatotoxicity if used with drugs that raise liver enzyme levels.	▪ Advise pt of this adverse effect. ▪ Monitor LFT values.
evening primrose oil	May lower the seizure threshold.	▪ Advise pt with seizure disorder to avoid herb.
hyssop **sage**	May counteract the antiseizure effects of anticonvulsants.	▪ Discourage use together. ▪ Monitor pt for loss of therapeutic effect of drug.
nettle	May increase sedative adverse effects. May increase risk of seizures.	▪ Advise pt of these effects. ▪ Advise pt with seizure disorder to avoid herb.
furosemide • Apo-Furosemide ◆, Furoside ◆, Lasix, Novosemide ◆, Uritol ◆		
agrimony bitter orange coriander dong quai fennel khella lovage motherwort Queen Anne's lace rosemary (topical) St. John's wort	Loop diuretics may increase photosensitivity, adding to the risk of sunburn or skin rash.	▪ Advise pt to wear a sunscreen or protective clothing during sun exposure.
aloe	May increase potassium-wasting effect of loop diuretics.	▪ Monitor potassium level. ▪ Monitor pt for signs and symptoms of hypokalemia.

Herb	Possible effects	Clinical tips
furosemide *(continued)*		
artichoke dandelion goldenseal	May enhance diuretic effects of drug.	▪ Discourage use together. ▪ Monitor pt for clinical effect. ▪ Monitor electrolytes.
dandelion uva-ursi	May decrease the effectiveness of the diuretic because of the sodium-sparing effect of herb.	▪ Monitor pt for therapeutic effect of med. ▪ Pt may want to avoid herb during diuretic therapy.
ginseng	Decreases effectiveness of the diuretic.	▪ Monitor pt for therapeutic effect of med. ▪ Pt may want to avoid herb during diuretic therapy.
gossypol	May potentiate the effects of the diuretic, including the increased risk of hypokalemia.	▪ Monitor potassium level. ▪ Pt may want to avoid herb during diuretic therapy.
licorice	May cause unexpectedly rapid potassium loss. However, deglycyrrhizinated licorice (DGL) shouldn't affect potassium level.	▪ Monitor potassium level. ▪ Monitor pt for signs and symptoms of hypokalemia, including muscle weakness, fatigue, nausea, vomiting, constipation, respiratory depression, and arrhythmias.
ganciclovir (DHPG) • Cytovene		
boneset **butterbur** **chaparral** **coltsfoot** **comfrey**	Contains pyrrolizidine alkaloids, which may be hepatotoxic.	▪ Monitor pt for signs and symptoms of liver damage, including abdominal pain, fever, malaise, jaundice, dark urine, clay-colored stools, and increased LFT values.
borage **fennel oil**	May decrease effectiveness of anticonvulsants.	▪ Advise pt with seizure disorder to avoid herb.

ginkgo **St. John's wort** **wormwood**		
echinacea	May increase hepatotoxicity if used with drugs that raise liver enzyme levels. May worsen HIV infection or AIDS.	▪ Advise pt with HIV infection or AIDS to avoid herb.
evening primrose oil	May lower the seizure threshold.	▪ Advise pt with seizure disorder to avoid herb.
milk thistle	Liver membrane stabilization and antioxidant effects of herb may protect against liver damage caused by various hepatotoxic drugs.	▪ May be used for therapeutic advantage. ▪ Monitor LFT values.
snakeroot	May increase risk of kidney problems because one component of snakeroot, aristolochic acid, has nephrotoxic properties.	▪ Discourage use of herb because of its toxic and carcinogenic potential.

gatifloxacin • Tequin

agrimony bitter orange coriander dong quai fennel khella lovage motherwort	May increase photosensitivity, adding to the risk of sunburn or skin rash.	▪ Advise pt to wear a sunscreen or protective clothing during sun exposure.

Herb	Possible effects	Clinical tips
gatifloxacin *(continued)*		
Queen Anne's lace rosemary (topical) St. John's wort	May increase photosensitivity, adding to the risk of sunburn or skin rash.	▪ Advise pt to wear a sunscreen or protective clothing during sun exposure.
Siberian ginseng	May enhance the effects of some antibiotics.	▪ May be used for therapeutic advantage.
gemfibrozil • Apo-Gemfibrozil ♦, Lopid		
boneset **butterbur** **chaparral** **coltsfoot** **comfrey**	Contains pyrrolizidine alkaloids, which may be hepatotoxic.	▪ Discourage use together. ▪ Monitor pt for signs and symptoms of liver damage, including abdominal pain, fever, malaise, jaundice, dark urine, clay-colored stools, and increased LFT values.
echinacea	May increase hepatotoxicity if used with drugs that raise liver enzyme levels.	▪ Advise pt of this adverse effect. ▪ Monitor LFT values.
garlic	May have additive lipid-lowering properties.	▪ May be used for therapeutic effect.
milk thistle	Liver membrane stabilization and antioxidant effects of herb may protect against liver damage caused by various hepatotoxic drugs.	▪ May be used for therapeutic advantage. ▪ Monitor LFT values.

gentamicin sulfate • Cidomycin ♦, Garamycin		
boneset **butterbur** **chaparral** **coltsfoot** **comfrey**	Contains pyrrolizidine alkaloids, which may be hepatotoxic.	▪ Monitor pt for signs and symptoms of liver damage, including abdominal pain, fever, malaise, jaundice, dark urine, clay-colored stools, and increased LFT values.
echinacea	May increase hepatotoxicity if used with drugs that raise liver enzyme levels.	▪ Advise pt of this adverse effect. ▪ Monitor LFT values.
milk thistle	Liver membrane stabilization and antioxidant effects of herb may protect against liver damage caused by various hepatotoxic drugs.	▪ Combination may be used for therapeutic advantage. ▪ Monitor LFT values.
snakeroot	May increase risk of kidney problems because one component of snakeroot, aristolochic acid, has nephrotoxic properties.	▪ Discourage use of herb because of its toxic and carcinogenic potential.

glipizide • Glucotrol, Glucotrol XL		
aloe bilberry leaf bitter melon bladderwrack burdock dandelion fenugreek garlic ginseng	Use together may improve blood sugar control, requiring a reduction of antidiabetic drugs. Herb may stimulate endogenous insulin release.	▪ Advise pt to consult health care provider before using herb. ▪ Monitor glucose level. ▪ Monitor pt for signs and symptoms of hypoglycemia, such as dizziness, diaphoresis, confusion, and tachycardia.

Interacting herbs in **bold type** indicate life-threatening interactions.

♦ Canadian

Herb	Possible effects	Clinical tips
glipizide *(continued)*		
basil bay bee pollen burdock ginkgo biloba ginseng glucomannan horehound marshmallow myrrh sage senega root yarrow	May affect glycemic control.	▪ Monitor glucose level. ▪ Monitor pt for signs and symptoms of hyperglycemia (fatigue, polyuria, polydipsia, wt loss, abdominal pain, altered mental status, tachycardia, hypotension, glucosuria, ketonuria) or hypoglycemia (dizziness, diaphoresis, confusion, tachycardia). ▪ Dosage adjustments may be needed.
echinacea	May increase hepatotoxicity if used with drugs that raise liver enzyme levels.	▪ Advise pt of this adverse effect. ▪ Monitor LFT values.
ma huang	May decrease hypoglycemic drug effect because of herb's hyperglycemic properties.	▪ Monitor glucose level. ▪ Monitor pt for signs and symptoms of hyperglycemia, including fatigue, polyuria, polydipsia, wt loss, abdominal pain, altered mental status, tachycardia, hypotension, glucosuria, and ketonuria.
glyburide • DiaBeta, Euglucon ♦, Glynase PresTab, Micronase		
aloe bilberry leaf	Use together may improve glycemic control, requiring reduction of antidiabetics.	▪ Advise pt to consult health care provider before using herb. ▪ Monitor glucose level.

bitter melon bladderwrack burdock dandelion fenugreek garlic ginseng	Herb may stimulate endogenous insulin release.	▪ Monitor pt for signs and symptoms of hypoglycemia, including dizziness, diaphoresis, confusion, and tachycardia.
basil bay bee pollen burdock ginkgo biloba ginseng glucomannan horehound marshmallow myrrh sage senega root yarrow	May affect glycemic control.	▪ Monitor glucose level. ▪ Monitor pt for signs and symptoms of hyperglycemia (fatigue, polyuria, polydipsia, wt loss, abdominal pain, altered mental status, tachycardia, hypotension, glucosuria, ketonuria) or hypoglycemia (dizziness, diaphoresis, confusion, tachycardia). ▪ Dosage adjustments may be needed.
echinacea	May increase hepatotoxicity if used with drug that raises liver enzyme levels.	▪ Advise pt of this adverse effect. ▪ Monitor LFT values.
ma huang	May decrease hypoglycemic drug effect because of herb's hyperglycemic properties.	▪ Monitor glucose level. ▪ Monitor pt for signs and symptoms of hyperglycemia, such as fatigue, polyuria, polydipsia, wt loss, abdominal pain, altered mental status, tachycardia, hypotension, glucosuria, and ketonuria.

Herb	Possible effects	Clinical tips
haloperidol • Apo-Haloperidol ◆, Haldol, Novo-Peridol ◆, Peridol ◆		
butterbur corkwood henbane jimsonweed	May increase anticholinergic adverse effects.	▪ Monitor pt for increased adverse effects, including headache, drowsiness, dizziness, confusion, irritability, tachycardia, mydriasis, dry mouth, constipation, urinary retention, and hot, dry skin.
ginseng ma huang	May increase CNS stimulant activity.	▪ Discourage use together.
milk thistle	Silymarin (contained in milk thistle) in combination with haloperidol causes a decrease in lipid peroxidation.	▪ Monitor LFT values. ▪ May be used for therapeutic advantage.
nutmeg	May cause a loss of symptom control or interfere with existing therapy for mental health.	▪ Discourage use together. ▪ Monitor pt for clinical effect.
heparin sodium • Hepalean ◆, Heparin Leo ◆, Heparin Sodium Injection		
angelica root anise arnica flower chamomile danshen devil's claw dong quai fenugreek garlic horse chestnut	May increase risk of bleeding because of coumarin or coumarin derivatives in herb. May inhibit platelet activation factor, increasing bleeding times in susceptible individuals.	▪ Monitor pt for signs and symptoms of increased bleeding, including bruising, petechiae, bleeding gums, epistaxis, prolonged bleeding after injury, melena, GI bleeding, hematuria, and hematemesis. ▪ Monitor results of hematologic studies and coagulation studies. ▪ Advise pt to consult health care provider before using herb.

Herb	Effect	Nursing considerations
licorice papain parsley passion flower red clover reishi mushroom rue sweet clover		
bilberry bromelain clove ginkgo biloba onion turmeric	May increase risk of bleeding because of coumarin or coumarin derivatives in herb or because of antiplatelet activity of herb.	▪ Monitor pt for signs and symptoms of increased bleeding, including bruising, petechiae, bleeding gums, epistaxis, prolonged bleeding after injury, melena, GI bleeding, hematuria, and hematemesis. ▪ Monitor results of hematologic studies and coagulation studies.
capsicum feverfew	Decreases platelet aggregation and increases fibrolytic activity, prolonging bleeding time.	▪ Monitor pt for signs and symptoms of increased bleeding, including bruising, petechiae, bleeding gums, epistaxis, prolonged bleeding after injury, melena, GI bleeding, hematuria, and hematemesis. ▪ Monitor results of hematologic studies and coagulation studies.
coenzyme Q10 ginseng St. John's wort	Antagonizes drug effects, resulting in a decreased INR.	▪ Monitor PT, PTT, and INR. ▪ Dosage adjustment may be needed.
echinacea	May increase bleeding time without elevating INR.	▪ Monitor pt for signs and symptoms of increased bleeding, including bruising, petechiae, bleeding

(continued)

Herb	Possible effects	Clinical tips
heparin sodium *(continued)*		
echinacea *(continued)*		gums, epistaxis, prolonged bleeding after injury, melena, GI bleeding, hematuria, and hematemesis.
ginger	Inhibits platelet aggregation by antagonizing thromboxane synthetase and enhancing prostacyclin, prolonging bleeding time.	▪ Monitor pt for signs and symptoms of increased bleeding, including bruising, petechiae, bleeding gums, epistaxis, prolonged bleeding after injury, melena, GI bleeding, hematuria, and hematemesis. ▪ Monitor results of hematologic studies and coagulation studies.
goldenseal	May counteract the anticoagulant effect of heparin.	▪ Monitor PTT and INR. ▪ Dosage adjustment may be needed.
grapeseed	Increases drug effects and INR because of tocopherol content of herb.	▪ Monitor pt for signs and symptoms of increased bleeding, including bruising, petechiae, bleeding gums, epistaxis, prolonged bleeding after injury, melena, GI bleeding, hematuria, and hematemesis. ▪ Monitor results of hematologic studies and coagulation studies.
green tea nettle	May cause antagonism because of vitamin K content in herb.	▪ Monitor pt for clinical effect. ▪ Monitor PT, PTT, and INR. ▪ Dosage adjustment may be needed.
meadowsweet white willow	May increase risk of bleeding because of salicylates in herb.	▪ Monitor pt for signs and symptoms of increased bleeding, including bruising, petechiae, bleeding gums, epistaxis, prolonged bleeding after injury, melena, GI bleeding, hematuria, and hematemesis.

Herb	Interaction	Management
		▪ Monitor results of hematologic studies and coagulation studies.
St. John's wort	May alter INR. Reduces the effectiveness of the anticoagulant, requiring increased dosage of drug.	▪ Monitor PT, PTT, and INR. ▪ Dosage adjustment may be needed.
hydrochlorothiazide • Apo-Hydro ◆, Diuchlor H ◆, Esidrix, Ezide, HydroDIURIL, Hydro-Par, Microzide, Neo-Codema ◆, Novo-Hydrazide ◆, Oretic, Urozide ◆		
agrimony bitter orange coriander dong quai fennel khella lovage motherwort Queen Anne's lace rosemary (topical) St. John's wort	May increase photosensitivity, adding to the risk of sunburn or skin rash.	▪ Advise pt to wear a sunscreen or protective clothing during sun exposure.
aloe buckthorn cascara sagrada senna	May cause additive potassium-wasting effect with thiazide diuretics.	▪ Monitor potassium level. ▪ Monitor pt for signs and symptoms of hypokalemia, including muscle weakness, fatigue, nausea, vomiting, constipation, respiratory depression, and arrhythmias.
artichoke dandelion	May potentiate the effects of the diuretic, including the increased risk of hypokalemia.	▪ Monitor potassium level. ▪ Discourage use of herb during diuretic therapy.

Herb	Possible effects	Clinical tips
hydrochlorothiazide *(continued)*		
goldenseal gossypol	May potentiate the effects of the diuretic, including the increased risk of hypokalemia.	▪ Monitor potassium level. ▪ Discourage use of herb during diuretic therapy.
ginseng	May decrease the diuretic effect.	▪ Monitor pt for clinical response.
licorice	May cause unexpectedly rapid potassium loss. However, deglycyrrhizinated licorice (DGL) shouldn't affect potassium level.	▪ Monitor potassium level. ▪ Monitor pt for signs and symptoms of hypokalemia, including muscle weakness, fatigue, nausea, vomiting, constipation, respiratory depression, and arrhythmias.
ibuprofen • Advil, Apo-Ibuprofen ◆, Genpril, Haltran, Ibuprin, Ibuprohm, Ibu-Tab, Medipren, Menadol, Motrin, Novo-Profen ◆, Nuprin, Rufen, Saleto-200, Trendar		
agrimony bitter orange coriander dong quai fennel khella lovage motherwort Queen Anne's lace rosemary (topical) St. John's wort	May increase photosensitivity, adding to risk of sunburn or skin rash.	▪ Advise pt to wear a sunscreen or protective clothing during sun exposure.
angelica root	May increase risk of bleeding because of	▪ Monitor pt for signs and symptoms of increased bleeding, in-

anise arnica flower bilberry bromelain capsicum chamomile clove danshen devil's claw dong quai echinacea fenugreek feverfew garlic ginger ginkgo biloba horse chestnut licorice onion papain parsley passion flower red clover reishi mushroom rue sweet clover turmeric	coumarin or coumarin derivatives in herb or because of antiplatelet activity of herb. May inhibit platelet activation factor, increasing bleeding times in susceptible individuals.	cluding bruising, petechiae, bleeding gums, epistaxis, prolonged bleeding after injury, melena, GI bleeding, hematuria, and hematemesis. ▪ Monitor results of hematologic studies and coagulation studies. ▪ Advise pt to consult health care provider before using herb.

Herb	Possible effects	Clinical tips
ibuprofen *(continued)*		
balsam of Peru **fumitory** **gossypol** **juniper** **monascus** **oak bark** **rue** **soapwort** **thunder god vine** **wild ginger** **wintergreen** **yohimbe**	Increases the risk of renal toxicity.	▪ Discourage use together. ▪ Monitor renal function tests.
boneset **butterbur** **chaparral** **coltsfoot** **comfrey**	Contains pyrrolizidine alkaloids, which may be hepatotoxic.	▪ Discourage use together. ▪ Monitor pt for signs and symptoms of liver damage, including abdominal pain, fever, malaise, jaundice, dark urine, clay-colored stools, and increased LFT values.
capsicum	Stimulates GI secretions to help protect against NSAID-induced GI irritation.	▪ May be used for therapeutic advantage.
Coffea arabica cola gossypol uva-ursi	May increase adverse GI effects.	▪ Advise pt of increased risk of adverse GI effects.

echinacea	May increase hepatotoxicity if used with drugs that raise liver enzyme levels.	▪ Advise pt of this adverse effect. ▪ Monitor LFT values.
meadowsweet white willow	May increase risk of bleeding because of salicylates in herb.	▪ Monitor pt for signs and symptoms of increased bleeding, including bruising, petechiae, bleeding gums, epistaxis, prolonged bleeding after injury, melena, GI bleeding, hematuria, and hematemesis. ▪ Monitor results of hematologic studies and coagulation studies.
milk thistle	Liver membrane stabilization and antioxidant effects of herb may protect against liver damage caused by various hepatotoxic drugs.	▪ Combination may be used for therapeutic advantage. ▪ Monitor LFT values.
wild yam	May decrease the anti-inflammatory effect of drug.	▪ Monitor pt for clinical effects.
imipramine • Apo-Imipramine ◆, Impril ◆, Norfranil, Novopramine ◆, Tipramine, Tofranil		
belladonna butterbur corkwood henbane jimsonweed	Increases anticholinergic effects.	▪ Monitor pt for increased adverse effects, including headache, dizziness, confusion, irritability, tachycardia, mydriasis, dry mouth, constipation, urinary retention, and hot, dry skin.
borage **fennel oil** **ginkgo** **wormwood**	May reduce the seizure threshold.	▪ Discourage use together. ▪ Monitor pt for seizure activity.

Herb	Possible effects	Clinical tips
imipramine *(continued)*		
capsicum catnip goldenseal **kava** lady's slipper lemon balm melatonin nettle passion flower sassafras skullcap valerian	May cause excessive physical depression, sedation, and impairment. Use of kava may cause coma.	▪ Monitor pt for signs and symptoms of increased CNS depression, including sedation, dizziness, drowsiness, ataxia, altered mental status, and respiratory depression.
evening primrose oil	May lower the seizure threshold and increase the risk of seizure activity.	▪ Discourage use together. ▪ Monitor pt for seizure activity.
SAMe **St. John's wort** **yohimbe**	May elevate serotonin level.	▪ Discourage use together. ▪ Monitor pt for signs and symptoms of serotonin syn, including nausea, hypotension, HTN, excitation, mental status changes, hyperpyrexia, and coma.
yohimbe	May cause HTN in pt taking TCA.	▪ Discourage use together. ▪ Monitor BP.
indinavir • Crixivan		
boneset **butterbur**	Contains pyrrolizidine alkaloids, which may be hepatotoxic.	▪ Discourage use together. ▪ Monitor pt for signs and symptoms of liver damage, including

Herb	Effect	Action
chaparral **coltsfoot** **comfrey**		abdominal pain, fever, malaise, jaundice, dark urine, clay-colored stools, and increased LFT values.
echinacea	May increase hepatotoxicity if used with drugs that raise liver enzyme levels. May exacerbate HIV by depressing CD+4 cells and increasing HIV replication.	▪ Advise pt of these effects. ▪ Discourage use together.
garlic	May cause severe GI toxicity resulting from concomitant use of ritonavir. May reduce the effectiveness of some drugs used for HIV infection.	▪ Discourage use together. ▪ Monitor pt for lack of therapeutic effect.
milk thistle	Liver membrane stabilization and antioxidant effects of herb may protect against liver damage caused by various hepatotoxic drugs.	▪ Combination may be used for therapeutic advantage. ▪ Monitor LFT values.
St. John's wort	Reduces blood level of indinavir by more than 50%; similar effects can be expected in other protease inhibitors.	▪ Discourage use together.

indomethacin • Apo-Indomethacin ◆, Indocid ◆, Indocid SR ◆, Indocin, Indocin SR, Novo-Methacin ◆

Herb	Effect	Action
agrimony bitter orange coriander dong quai fennel	May increase photosensitivity, adding to risk of sunburn or skin rash.	▪ Advise pt to wear a sunscreen or protective clothing during sun exposure.

Herb	Possible effects	Clinical tips
indomethacin *(continued)*		
khella lovage motherwort Queen Anne's lace rosemary (topical) St. John's wort	May increase photosensitivity, adding to risk of sunburn or skin rash.	▪ Advise pt to wear a sunscreen or protective clothing during sun exposure.
angelica root anise arnica flower bilberry bromelain capsicum chamomile clove danshen devil's claw dong quai echinacea fenugreek feverfew garlic ginger	May increase risk of bleeding because of coumarin or coumarin derivatives in herb or because of antiplatelet activity of herb. May inhibit platelet activation factor, increasing bleeding times in susceptible individuals.	▪ Monitor pt for signs and symptoms of increased bleeding, including bruising, petechiae, bleeding gums, epistaxis, prolonged bleeding after injury, melena, GI bleeding, hematuria, and hematemesis. ▪ Monitor results of hematologic studies and coagulation studies. ▪ Advise pt to consult health care provider before using herb.

ginkgo biloba horse chestnut licorice onion papain parsley passion flower red clover reishi mush- room rue sweet clover turmeric		
balsam of Peru **fumitory** **gossypol** **juniper** **monascus** **oak bark** **rue** **soapwort** **thunder god vine** **wild ginger** **wintergreen** **yohimbe**	Increases the risk of renal toxicity.	▪ Discourage use together. ▪ Monitor renal function tests.

Herb	Possible effects	Clinical tips
indomethacin *(continued)*		
capsicum	Stimulates GI secretions to help protect against NSAID-induced GI irritation.	▪ May be used for therapeutic advantage.
Coffea arabica cola gossypol uva-ursi	May increase adverse GI effects.	▪ Advise pt of increased risk of adverse GI effects.
meadowsweet white willow	May increase risk of bleeding because of salicylates in this herb.	▪ Monitor pt for signs and symptoms of increased bleeding, including bruising, petechiae, bleeding gums, epistaxis, prolonged bleeding after injury, melena, GI bleeding, hematuria, and hematemesis. ▪ Monitor results of hematologic studies and coagulation studies.
snakeroot	May increase risk of kidney problems because one component of snakeroot, aristolochic acid, has nephrotoxic properties.	▪ Discourage use of herb because of its toxic and carcinogenic potential.
wild yam	May decrease the anti-inflammatory effect of drug.	▪ Monitor pt for lack of therapeutic effect.
insulin injection (regular insulin) • Humulin-R, Humulin-R (concentrated) Regular U-500, Novolin R, Novolin R PenFill, Regular Iletin I, Regular Iletin II, Regular Purified Pork Insulin, Velosulin Human BR ◆		
aloe bilberry leaf bitter melon	Use together may improve glycemic control, requiring reduction of antidiabetics. May stimulate endogenous insulin release.	▪ Advise pt to consult health care provider before using herb. ▪ Monitor glucose level. ▪ Monitor pt for signs and symptoms of hypoglycemia, such as

bladderwrack burdock dandelion fenugreek garlic ginseng		dizziness, diaphoresis, confusion, and tachycardia.
aloe **buckthorn** **cascara sagrada** **Chinese rhubarb** **frangula** **guarana** **licorice** **senna**	May cause a change in cardiac rhythm and increase the potential for arrhythmias because herb use causes hypokalemia.	▪ Monitor potassium level. ▪ Monitor pt for signs and symptoms of hypokalemia, including muscle weakness, fatigue, nausea, vomiting, constipation, respiratory depression, and arrhythmias.
angelica root buchu juniper ma huang	Decreases hypoglycemic effect because of the hyperglycemia caused by herb.	▪ Monitor glucose level. ▪ Monitor pt for signs and symptoms of hyperglycemia, such as fatigue, polyuria, polydipsia, wt loss, abdominal pain, altered mental status, tachycardia, hypotension, glucosuria, and ketonuria.
basil bay bee pollen burdock ginkgo biloba ginseng	May affect glycemic control.	▪ Monitor glucose level. ▪ Monitor pt for signs and symptoms of hyperglycemia (fatigue, polyuria, polydipsia, wt loss, abdominal pain, altered mental status, tachycardia, hypotension, glucosuria, ketonuria) or hypoglycemia (dizziness, diaphoresis, confusion, tachycardia). ▪ Dosage adjustments may be needed.

Herb	Possible effects	Clinical tips
insulin injection (regular insulin) *(continued)*		
glucomannan horehound marshmallow myrrh sage senega root yarrow	May affect glycemic control.	▪ Monitor glucose level. ▪ Monitor pt for signs and symptoms of hyperglycemia (fatigue, polyuria, polydipsia, wt loss, abdominal pain, altered mental status, tachycardia, hypotension, glucosuria, ketonuria) or hypoglycemia (dizziness, diaphoresis, confusion, tachycardia). ▪ Dosage adjustments may be needed.
iron • DexFerrum, InFeD		
black cohosh chamomile feverfew gossypol hawthorn nettle plantain saw palmetto St. John's wort valerian	May decrease iron absorption because herb contains tannins; tannin-iron complex may form.	▪ Monitor pt for adequate response to iron therapy.
oregano	May reduce iron absorption.	▪ Advise pt to separate administration times by > 2 h when given with iron suppl or iron-containing foods.
isoniazid (INH) • Isotamine ◆, Laniazid, Nydrazid, PMS-Isoniazid ◆		
boneset **butterbur**	Contains pyrrolizidine alkaloids, which may be hepatotoxic.	▪ Monitor pt for signs and symptoms of liver damage, including abdominal pain, fever, malaise, jaundice, dark urine, clay-

chaparral **coltsfoot** **comfrey**		
echinacea	May increase hepatotoxicity if used with drugs that raise liver enzyme levels. May exacerbate tuberculosis.	▪ Adv... ▪ Monitor L...
licorice	Glycyrrhizin obtained from licorice has been used with INH to treat tuberculosis.	▪ Advise pt to consu...
milk thistle	Liver membrane stabilization and antioxidant effects of herb may protect against liver damage caused by various hepatotoxic drugs.	▪ May be used for therapeutic adva... ▪ Monitor LFT values.

ective clothing during sun

isradipine • DynaCirc

black cohosh	May increase peripheral vasodilation, resulting in hypotension.	▪ Monitor BP closely. ▪ Dosage adjustment may be needed.
ginger	May increase calcium uptake by the myocardium, leading to altered drug effects.	▪ Advise pt of this effect. ▪ Monitor pt for clinical response.
goldenseal	May interfere with drug's action because the alkaloids of herb have hypertensive properties.	▪ Monitor pt for clinical effect. ▪ Monitor BP.
licorice	May increase sodium, chloride, and H_20 retention, resulting in BP increase.	▪ Monitor BP.

Herb	Possible effects	Clinical tips
isradipine *(continued)*		
yohimbe bark	May cause a decrease in drug effect because of hypertensive effects of herb.	▪ Monitor BP closely. ▪ Dosage adjustment may be needed.
ketoconazole • Nizoral		
boneset **butterbur** **chaparral** **coltsfoot** **comfrey**	Contains pyrrolizidine alkaloids, which may be hepatotoxic.	▪ Monitor pt for signs and symptoms of liver damage, including abdominal pain, fever, malaise, jaundice, dark urine, clay-colored stools, and increased LFT values.
echinacea	May increase hepatotoxicity if used with drugs that raise liver enzyme levels.	▪ Advise pt of this adverse effect. ▪ Monitor LFT values.
milk thistle	Liver membrane stabilization and antioxidant effects of herb may protect against liver damage caused by various hepatotoxic drugs.	▪ Combination may be used for therapeutic advantage. ▪ Monitor LFT values.
yew	Inhibits ketoconazole metabolism.	▪ Discourage use together. ▪ Advise pt of this effect.
ketoprofen • Actron, Apo-Keto ◆, Novo-Keto-EC ◆, Orudis, Orudis E ◆, Orudis KT, Orudis SR ◆, Oruvail, Rhodis ◆, Rhodis-EC ◆		
agrimony bitter orange coriander dong quai	May increase photosensitivity, adding to risk of sunburn and skin rash.	▪ Advise pt to wear a sunscr[illegible] exposure.

fennel khella lovage motherwort Queen Anne's lace rosemary (topical) St. John's wort		
angelica root anise arnica flower bilberry bromelain capsicum chamomile clove danshen devil's claw dong quai echinacea fenugreek feverfew garlic ginger ginkgo biloba horse chestnut licorice	May increase risk of bleeding because of coumarin or coumarin derivatives in herb or because of antiplatelet activity of herb. May inhibit platelet activation factor, increasing bleeding times in susceptible individuals.	▪ Monitor pt for signs and symptoms of increased bleeding, including bruising, petechiae, bleeding gums, epistaxis, prolonged bleeding after injury, melena, GI bleeding, hematuria, and hematemesis. ▪ Monitor results of hematologic studies and coagulation studies. ▪ Advise pt to consult health care provider before using herb.

Herb	Possible effects	Clinical tips
ketoprofen *(continued)*		
onion papain parsley passion flower red clover reishi mushroom rue sweet clover turmeric	May increase risk of bleeding because of coumarin or coumarin derivatives in herb or because of antiplatelet activity of herb. May inhibit platelet activation factor, increasing bleeding times in susceptible individuals.	▪ Monitor pt for signs and symptoms of increased bleeding, including bruising, petechiae, bleeding gums, epistaxis, prolonged bleeding after injury, melena, GI bleeding, hematuria, and hematemesis. ▪ Monitor results of hematologic studies and coagulation studies. ▪ Advise pt to consult health care provider before using herb.
balsam of Peru **fumitory** **gossypol** **juniper** **monascus** **oak bark** **rue** **soapwort** **thunder god vine** **wild ginger** **wintergreen** **yohimbe**	Increases the risk of renal toxicity.	▪ Discourage use together. ▪ Monitor renal function tests.
boneset **butterbur**	Contains pyrrolizidine alkaloids, which may be hepatotoxic.	▪ Discourage use together. ▪ Monitor pt for signs and symptoms of liver damage, including

chaparral **coltsfoot** **comfrey**		abdominal pain, fever, malaise, jaundice, dark urine, clay-colored stools, and increased LFT values.
capsicum	Stimulates GI secretions to help protect against NSAID-induced GI irritation.	▪ May be used for therapeutic advantage.
Coffea arabica cola gossypol uva-ursi	May increase adverse GI effects.	▪ Advise pt of increased risk of adverse GI effects.
echinacea	May increase hepatotoxicity if used with drugs that raise liver enzyme levels.	▪ Advise pt of this adverse effect. ▪ Monitor LFT values.
meadowsweet white willow	May increase risk of bleeding because of salicylates in the herbs.	▪ Monitor pt for signs and symptoms of increased bleeding, including bruising, petechiae, bleeding gums, epistaxis, prolonged bleeding after injury, melena, GI bleeding, hematuria, and hematemesis. ▪ Monitor results of hematologic studies and coagulation studies.
milk thistle	Liver membrane stabilization and antioxidant effects of herb may protect against liver damage caused by various hepatotoxic drugs.	▪ Combination may be used for therapeutic advantage. ▪ Monitor LFT values.
snakeroot	May increase risk of kidney problems because one component of herb, aristolochic acid, has nephrotoxic properties.	▪ Discourage use of herb because of its toxic and carcinogenic potential.

Interacting herbs in **bold type** indicate life-threatening interactions.

◆ Canadian

Herb	Possible effects	Clinical tips
ketoprofen *(continued)*		
wild yam	May decrease the anti-inflammatory effect of drug.	▪ Monitor pt for clinical effects.
ketorolac tromethamine • Toradol		
agrimony bitter orange coriander dong quai fennel khella lovage motherwort Queen Anne's lace rosemary (topical) St. John's wort	May increase photosensitivity, adding to risk of sunburn or skin rash.	▪ Advise pt to wear a sunscreen or protective clothing during sun exposure.
angelica root anise arnica flower bilberry bromelain capsicum chamomile clove	May increase risk of bleeding because of coumarin or coumarin derivatives in herb or because of antiplatelet activity of herb. May inhibit platelet activation factor, increasing bleeding times in susceptible individuals.	▪ Monitor pt for signs and symptoms of increased bleeding, including bruising, petechiae, bleeding gums, epistaxis, prolonged bleeding after injury, melena, GI bleeding, hematuria, and hematemesis. ▪ Monitor results of hematologic studies and coagulation studies. ▪ Advise pt to consult health care provider before using herb.

danshen devil's claw dong quai echinacea fenugreek feverfew garlic ginger ginkgo biloba horse chestnut licorice onion papain parsley passion flower red clover reishi mushroom rue sweet clover turmeric		
balsam of Peru **fumitory** **gossypol** **juniper** **monascus** **oak bark** **rue**	Increases the risk of renal toxicity.	▪ Discourage use together. ▪ Monitor renal function tests.

Herb	Possible effects	Clinical tips
ketorolac tromethamine *(continued)*		
soapwort **thunder god vine** **wild ginger** **wintergreen** **yohimbe**	Increases the risk of renal toxicity.	▪ Discourage use together. ▪ Monitor renal function tests.
boneset **butterbur** **chaparral** **coltsfoot** **comfrey**	Contains pyrrolizidine alkaloids, which may be hepatotoxic.	▪ Discourage use together. ▪ Monitor pt for signs and symptoms of liver damage, including abdominal pain, fever, malaise, jaundice, dark urine, clay-colored stools, and increased LFT values.
capsicum	Stimulates GI secretions to help protect against NSAID-induced GI irritation.	▪ May be used for therapeutic advantage.
Coffea arabica cola gossypol uva-ursi	May increase adverse GI effects.	▪ Advise pt of increased risk of adverse GI effects.
echinacea	May increase hepatotoxicity if used with drugs that raise liver enzyme levels.	▪ Advise pt of this adverse effect. ▪ Monitor LFT values.
meadowsweet white willow	May increase risk of bleeding because of salicylates in the herbs.	▪ Monitor pt for signs and symptoms of increased bleeding, including bruising, petechiae, bleeding gums, epistaxis, prolonged bleeding after injury, melena, GI bleeding, hematuria, and hematemesis.

		▪ Monitor results of hematologic studies and coagulation studies.
milk thistle	Liver membrane stabilization and antioxidant effects of herb may protect against liver damage caused by various hepatotoxic drugs.	▪ Combination may be used for therapeutic advantage. ▪ Monitor LFT values.
snakeroot	May increase risk of kidney problems because one component of snakeroot, aristolochic acid, has nephrotoxic properties.	▪ Discourage use of herb because of its toxic and carcinogenic potential.
wild yam	May decrease the anti-inflammatory effect of drug.	▪ Monitor pt for clinical effects.
labetalol • Normodyne, Trandate		
black cohosh	May increase peripheral vasodilation, resulting in hypotension.	▪ Monitor BP closely. ▪ Dosage adjustment may be needed.
ginger	May antagonize antihypertensive effect.	▪ Monitor BP.
goldenseal	May interfere with drug's action because the alkaloids of herb have hypertensive properties.	▪ Monitor pt for clinical effect. ▪ Monitor BP.
licorice	May increase sodium, chloride, and H_20 retention, resulting in BP increase.	▪ Monitor BP.
saw palmetto	May have an additive alpha adrenergic blocking effect when combined with alpha blockers.	▪ Monitor pt for hypotension. ▪ Dosage adjustment may be needed.

Herb	Possible effects	Clinical tips
labetalol *(continued)*		
yohimbe bark	May cause a decrease in drug effect because of hypertensive effects of herb.	▪ Advise pt of this effect. ▪ Monitor BP closely.
lamivudine • Epivir, Epivir-HBV		
boneset **butterbur** **chaparral** **coltsfoot** **comfrey**	Contains pyrrolizidine alkaloids, which may be hepatotoxic.	▪ Monitor pt for signs and symptoms of liver damage, including abdominal pain, fever, malaise, jaundice, dark urine, clay-colored stools, and increased LFT values.
echinacea	May increase hepatotoxicity if used with drugs that raise liver enzyme levels. May exacerbate HIV disease by depressing CD+4 cells and increasing HIV replication.	▪ Discourage use together. ▪ Advise pt of these adverse effects.
milk thistle	Liver membrane stabilization and antioxidant effects of herb may protect against liver damage caused by various hepatotoxic drugs.	▪ Combination may be used for therapeutic advantage. ▪ Monitor LFT values.
lansoprazole •Prevacid		
agrimony bitter orange coriander dong quai fennel khella	May increase photosensitivity, adding to the risk of sunburn or skin rash.	▪ Advise pt to wear a sunscreen or protective clothing during sun exposure.

Herb	Interaction	Action
lovage motherwort Queen Anne's lace rosemary (topical) St. John's wort		
blessed thistle bogbean capsicum ginger goldenseal mustard	May decrease drug effectiveness because of increased acid secretion caused by herb.	▪ Advise pt of this effect. ▪ Monitor pt for therapeutic response.
levalbuterol hydrochloride • Xopenex		
capsicum ginseng ma huang Scotch broom yohimbe	May increase adverse effects of drug.	▪ Monitor pt for increased adverse effects such as HTN, tachycardia, palpitations, and CNS stimulant effects.
licorice root	May increase BP and heart rate.	▪ Monitor vital signs and ECG.
St. John's wort	May have MAO inhibitor properties.	▪ May increase vascular response. ▪ Monitor vital signs and ECG closely.
levetiracetam • Keppra		
borage **fennel oil**	May decrease effectiveness of anticonvulsants.	▪ Discourage use together.

Herb	Possible effects	Clinical tips
levetiracetam *(continued)*		
ginkgo **St. John's wort** **wormwood**	May decrease effectiveness of anticonvulsants.	▪ Discourage use together.
evening primrose oil	May lower the seizure threshold.	▪ Discourage use together. ▪ Monitor pt for loss of therapeutic effect of drug.
hyssop **sage**	May counteract the antiseizure effects of anticonvulsants.	▪ Discourage use together. ▪ Monitor pt for loss of therapeutic effect of drug.
nettle	May increase sedative adverse effects. May increase risk of seizures.	▪ Discourage use together. ▪ Monitor pt for loss of therapeutic effect of drug and increased sedation.
levodopa-carbidopa • Sinemet, Sinemet CR		
boneset **butterbur** **chaparral** **coltsfoot** **comfrey**	Contains pyrrolizidine alkaloids, which may be hepatotoxic.	▪ Monitor pt for signs and symptoms of liver damage, including abdominal pain, fever, malaise, jaundice, dark urine, clay-colored stools, and increased LFT values.
echinacea	May increase hepatotoxicity if used with drugs that raise liver enzyme levels.	▪ Advise pt of this adverse effect. ▪ Monitor LFT values.
5-HTP	May cause skin changes similar to those that occur in scleroderma.	▪ Discourage use together. ▪ Advise pt of this effect.
kava	May interfere with drug's action as well as	▪ Discourage use together.

Herb	Effect	Management
	that of natural dopamine. May worsen symptoms of Parkinson's disease.	▪ Monitor pt for therapeutic clinical response.
milk thistle	Liver membrane stabilization and antioxidant effects of herb may protect against liver damage caused by various hepatotoxic drugs.	▪ Combination may be used for therapeutic advantage. ▪ Monitor LFT values.
rauwolfia	May decrease drug effects. May increase extrapyramidal symptoms.	▪ Discourage use together. ▪ Monitor pt for increased adverse effect.
SAMe	May interfere with the action of levodopa.	▪ Advise pt of this effect. ▪ Monitor pt for clinical response.
levofloxacin • Levaquin		
agrimony bitter orange coriander dong quai fennel khella lovage motherwort Queen Anne's lace rosemary (topical) St. John's wort	Fluoroquinolone antibiotics may increase photosensitivity, adding to the risk of sunburn or rash.	▪ Advise pt to wear a sunscreen or protective clothing during sun exposure.

Herb	Possible effects	Clinical tips
levofloxacin *(continued)*		
fennel	May reduce blood level of drug, possibly impairing its effectiveness. Herb might be expected to interfere similarly with other fluoroquinolone antibiotics.	▪ Advise pt to avoid, if possible, use of herb with this drug and other fluoroquinolone antibiotics. Otherwise, advise pt to separate use by 2 h to reduce the potential for an interaction. Emphasize that this may not eliminate the risk of interaction.
levothyroxine • Eltroxin ◆, Levo-T, Levothroid, Levoxine, Levoxyl, Synthroid		
bugleweed	May have antithyrotropic activity. May inhibit peripheral deiodination of T_4.	▪ Discourage pt with hypothyroidism from using herb.
capsicum ma huang Scotch broom yohimbe	May increase catecholamine levels.	▪ Monitor pt for increased adverse effects, including tachycardia, HTN, and arrhythmias.
guggal	May alter the effects of thyroid drugs because herb stimulates the thyroid gland.	▪ Discourage use together.
kelp	May cause hyperthyroidism because of the iodine content in herb.	▪ Discourage use together. ▪ Dosage adjustment may be needed if used together.
shepherd's purse	Allyl isothiocyanate may interfere with thyroid therapy.	▪ Monitor thyroid function.
lisinopril • Prinivil, Zestril		
agrimony bitter orange coriander dong quai	ACE inhibitors may increase photosensitivity, adding to the risk of sunburn or skin rash.	▪ Advise pt to wear a sunscreen or protective clothing during sun exposure.

fennel khella lovage motherwort Queen Anne's lace rosemary (topical) St. John's wort		
black catechu	May increase hypotensive effect of herb.	▪ Monitor BP. ▪ Dosage adjustment may be needed.
black cohosh	May increase peripheral vasodilation, resulting in hypotension.	▪ Monitor BP closely. ▪ Dosage adjustment may be needed.
capsaicin	May increase risk of cough.	▪ Discourage use to avoid increased risk of cough.
ginger	May antagonize antihypertensive effect.	▪ Monitor BP closely. ▪ Dosage adjustment may be needed.
goldenseal	May interfere with drug's action because the alkaloids of herb have hypertensive properties.	▪ Monitor pt for clinical effect. ▪ Monitor BP.
licorice	May cause sodium retention and increase BP, interfering with the therapeutic effects of ACE inhibitors.	▪ Advise pt of this interaction. ▪ Monitor BP.
yohimbe bark	May decrease drug effects because of hypertensive effects of herb.	▪ Monitor BP closely. ▪ Dosage adjustment may be needed.

Herb	Possible effects	Clinical tips
lithium • Carbolith ◆, Duralith ◆, Eskalith, Eskalith CR, Lithane, Lithizine ◆, Lithobid, Lithonate, Lithotabs		
angelica root **buchu** **dandelion** **juniper**	May increase the effects of lithium. May cause lithium toxicity.	▪ Monitor lithium level. ▪ Monitor pt for increased adverse effects.
green tea **guarana**	May cause an increased lithium level if caffeine (contained in herb) is abruptly stopped.	▪ Monitor lithium level. ▪ Monitor pt for signs and symptoms of lithium toxicity, including sedation, confusion, tremors, muscle stiffness, increased deep tendon reflexes, visual changes, and nystagmus. ▪ Dosage adjustment may be needed.
ispaghula plantain	May inhibit absorption of drug in the GI tract, decreasing serum concentration.	▪ Monitor pt for lack or loss of therapeutic effect. ▪ Discourage use together.
snakeroot	May increase risk of kidney problems because one component of snakeroot, aristolochic acid, has nephrotoxic properties.	▪ Discourage use of herb because of its toxic and carcinogenic potential.
loratadine • Claritin, Claritin Reditabs, Claritin Syrup		
agrimony bitter orange coriander dong quai fennel khella lovage motherwort	May increase photosensitivity, adding to risk of sunburn or skin rash.	▪ Advise pt to wear a sunscreen or protective clothing during sun exposure.

Herb	Effect	Nursing considerations
Queen Anne's lace rosemary (topical) St. John's wort		
butterbur corkwood henbane jimsonweed	Increases anticholinergic effects.	▪ Monitor pt for increased adverse effects, including headache, drowsiness, dizziness, confusion, irritability, tachycardia, mydriasis, dry mouth, constipation, urinary retention, and hot, dry skin.
licorice	May prolong the QT interval. May cause additive effects.	▪ Advise pt of this effect. ▪ Monitor pt for adverse cardiac events such as arrhythmias.
lorazepam • Apo-Lorazepam ◆, Ativan, Lorazepam Intensol, Novo-Lorazem ◆		
capsicum catnip goldenseal **kava** lady's slipper lemon balm melatonin nettle passion flower sassafras skullcap valerian	May cause excessive physical depression, sedation, and impairment. Use of kava may cause coma.	▪ Discourage use together. ▪ Monitor pt for signs and symptoms of increased CNS depression, including sedation, drowsiness, dizziness, ataxia, altered mental status, and respiratory depression.
linden	May increase side effects of benzodiazepines because herb contains similar components.	▪ Advise pt not to take excessive amt of herb.

Herb	Possible effects	Clinical tips
lovastatin • Mevacor		
boneset **butterbur** **chaparral** **coltsfoot** **comfrey**	Contains pyrrolizidine alkaloids, which may be hepatotoxic.	▪ Discourage use together. ▪ Monitor pt for signs and symptoms of liver damage, including abdominal pain, fever, malaise, jaundice, dark urine, clay-colored stools, and increased LFT values.
echinacea	May increase hepatotoxicity if used with drugs that raise liver enzyme levels.	▪ Monitor LFT values.
garlic	May have additive lipid-lowering properties.	▪ May be used for therapeutic advantage.
milk thistle	Liver membrane stabilization and antioxidant effects of herb may protect against liver damage caused by various hepatotoxic drugs.	▪ Combination may be used for therapeutic advantage. ▪ Monitor LFT values.
pectin	May decrease the effectiveness of HMG-CoA reductase inhibitors.	▪ Discourage use together. ▪ Monitor pt for clinical response.
red yeast rice	Contains similar components to those of statin drugs, increasing the risk of adverse events or toxicity.	▪ Discourage use together if possible. Monitor pt for signs and symptoms of increased adverse effects such as myopathy and rhabdomyolysis (increased serum creatinine kinase level, muscle aches, weakness) or increased LFT values.
St. John's wort	May decrease blood levels of various drugs in the statin family.	▪ Monitor pt for clinical response.

meloxicam • Mobic

Herb	Interaction	Nursing considerations
angelica root anise bilberry borage seed oil danshen devil's claw dong quai echinacea feverfew garlic ginger ginkgo biloba horse chestnut licorice passion flower red clover	May increase risk of bleeding because of coumarin or coumarin derivatives in the herb or because of the herb's antiplatelet activity.	▪ Monitor pt for signs and symptoms of increased bleeding, including bruising, petechiae, bleeding gums, epistaxis, prolonged bleeding after injury, melena, GI bleeding, hematuria, and hematemesis. ▪ Monitor results of hematologic studies and coagulation studies. ▪ Advise pt to consult health care provider before using herb.
bitter melon **fenugreek** **skullcap** **woundwort** **yerba maté**	May cause hepatotoxicity.	▪ Monitor LFT values. ▪ Signs and symptoms of liver damage include abdominal pain, fever, malaise, jaundice, dark urine, clay-colored stools, and increased LFT values. ▪ Discourage use together.
boneset **butterbur** **chaparral**	Contains pyrrolizidine alkaloids, which may be hepatotoxic.	▪ Discourage use together. ▪ Signs and symptoms of liver damage include abdominal pain, fever, malaise, jaundice, dark urine, *(continued)*

Herb	Possible effects	Clinical tips
meloxicam *(continued)*		
coltsfoot **comfrey**		clay-colored stools, and increased LFT values.
echinacea	May increase hepatotoxicity if used with drugs that elevate liver enzyme levels.	▪ Advise pt of this adverse effect. ▪ Monitor LFT values.
fumitory **gossypol** **juniper** **oak bark** **wild ginger** **wintergreen** **yohimbe**	May increase risk of nephrotoxicity or RF.	▪ Advise pt about herb's nephrotoxic potential. ▪ Monitor results of renal function studies.
kava	May increase risk of hepatic adverse reactions, such as cirrhosis, hepatitis, or liver failure.	▪ Discourage use together. ▪ Monitor LFT values. ▪ Advise pt to report signs and symptoms of liver problems to health care provider.
meadowsweet white willow	May increase risk of bleeding because of salicylates in the herb.	▪ Monitor pt for signs and symptoms of increased bleeding, including bruising, petechiae, bleeding gums, epistaxis, prolonged bleeding after injury, melena, GI bleeding, hematuria, and hematemesis. ▪ Monitor results of hematologic studies and coagulation studies.
snakeroot	May increase risk of renal problems because one component of snakeroot, aristolochic	▪ Discourage use together because of herb's toxic and carcinogenic potential.

acid, has nephrotoxic properties.

metformin • Glucophage		
aloe bilberry leaf bitter melon bladderwrack burdock dandelion fenugreek garlic ginseng goat's rue gymnema	May improve glucose control, requiring a reduction of antidiabetics. May stimulate endogenous insulin release.	▪ Advise pt to consult health care provider before using herb. ▪ Monitor glucose level. ▪ Monitor pt for signs and symptoms of hypoglycemia, such as dizziness, diaphoresis, confusion, and tachycardia.
angelica broom buchu juniper ma huang	May decrease drug's hypoglycemic effect because of herbs' hyperglycemic properties.	▪ Monitor glucose level. ▪ Monitor pt for signs and symptoms of hyperglycemia, such as fatigue, polyuria, altered mental status, glucosuria, and ketonuria.
balsam of Peru **fumitory** **gossypol** **juniper** **monascus** **oak bark** **rue** **soapwort**	May increase risk of nephrotoxicity or RF.	▪ Monitor pt for signs and symptoms of lactic acidosis (malaise, myalgia, respiratory distress, increased somnolence, abdominal discomfort, hypothermia, hypotension, and bradyarrhythmias), which can cause renal dysfunction.

Herb	Possible effects	Clinical tips
metformin *(continued)*		
thunder god vine **wild ginger** **wintergreen** **yohimbe**	May increase risk of nephrotoxicity or RF.	▪ Monitor pt for signs and symptoms of lactic acidosis (malaise, myalgia, respiratory distress, increased somnolence, abdominal discomfort, hypothermia, hypotension, and bradyarrhythmias), which can cause renal dysfunction.
basil bay bee pollen burdock ginkgo biloba ginseng glucomannan horehound marshmallow myrrh sage senega root yarrow	May disrupt antidiabetic therapy and affect glycemic control.	▪ Monitor glucose level. ▪ Monitor pt for signs and symptoms of hyperglycemia (fatigue, polyuria, altered mental status, glucosuria, and ketonuria) or hypoglycemia (dizziness, diaphoresis, confusion, tachycardia).
snakeroot	May increase risk of renal problems because one component of snakeroot, aristolochic acid, has nephrotoxic properties.	▪ Discourage use together because of herb's toxic and carcinogenic potential.
methotrexate • Folex, Folex PFS, Rheumatrex		
agrimony bitter orange	May increase photosensitivity, adding to risk of sunburn or rash.	▪ Advise pt to wear sunscreen or protective clothing during sun exposure.

celery seed coriander dong quai fennel khella lovage motherwort Queen Anne's lace rosemary (topical) St. John's wort		
bitter melon **fenugreek** **skullcap** **woundwort** **yerba maté**	May cause hepatotoxicity.	▪ Monitor LFT values. ▪ Signs and symptoms of liver damage include abdominal pain, fever, malaise, jaundice, dark urine, clay-colored stools, and increased LFT values.
boneset **butterbur** **chaparral** **coltsfoot** **comfrey**	Contains pyrrolizidine alkaloids, which may be hepatotoxic.	▪ Discourage use together. ▪ Signs and symptoms of liver damage include abdominal pain, fever, malaise, jaundice, dark urine, clay-colored stools, and increased LFT values.
echinacea	May increase hepatotoxicity if used with drugs that elevate liver enzyme levels.	▪ Advise pt of this adverse effect. ▪ Monitor LFT values.
fumitory **gossypol**	May increase risk of nephrotoxicity or RF.	▪ Advise pt of herb's nephrotoxic potential. ▪ Monitor results of renal function studies.

Herb	Possible effects	Clinical tips
methotrexate *(continued)*		
juniper **oak bark** **wild ginger** **wintergreen** **yohimbe**	May increase risk of nephrotoxicity or RF.	▪ Advise pt of herb's nephrotoxic potential. ▪ Monitor results of renal function studies.
kava	May increase risk of hepatic adverse reactions, such as cirrhosis, hepatitis, or liver failure.	▪ Discourage use together. ▪ Monitor LFT values. ▪ Advise pt to report signs and symptoms of liver problems to health care provider.
snakeroot	May increase risk of renal problems because one component of snakeroot, aristolochic acid, has nephrotoxic properties.	▪ Discourage use together because of herb's toxic and carcinogenic potential.
methyldopa • Aldomet, Apo-Methyldopa ♦, Dopamet ♦, Novomedopa ♦, Nu-Medopa ♦		
bitter melon **fenugreek** **skullcap** **woundwort** **yerba maté**	May cause hepatotoxicity.	▪ Monitor LFT values. ▪ Signs and symptoms of liver damage include abdominal pain, fever, malaise, jaundice, dark urine, clay-colored stools, and increased LFT values.
black cohosh	May increase peripheral vasodilation, resulting in hypotension.	▪ Monitor BP closely. ▪ Dosage adjustment may be needed.
boneset **butterbur**	Contains pyrrolizidine alkaloids, which may be hepatotoxic.	▪ Signs and symptoms of liver damage include abdominal pain, fever, malaise, jaundice, dark urine, clay-colored stools, and

Herb	Interaction	Action
chaparral **coltsfoot** **comfrey**		increased LFT values.
echinacea	May increase hepatotoxicity if used with drugs that elevate liver enzyme levels.	▪ Advise pt of this adverse effect. ▪ Monitor LFT values.
kava	May increase risk of hepatic adverse reactions, such as cirrhosis, hepatitis, or liver failure.	▪ Discourage use together. ▪ Monitor LFT values. ▪ Advise pt to report signs and symptoms of liver problems to health care provider.
licorice	May increase sodium, chloride, and H_2O retention, resulting in BP increase.	▪ Monitor BP.
methylphenidate • Concerta, Metadate CD, Metadate ER, Methylin, PMS-Methylphenidate ◆, Ritalin		
boldo	Stimulates the CNS, causing exaggerated reflexes, incoordination, and seizures.	▪ Discourage use together. ▪ Watch for CNS overstimulation.
borage **evening primrose oil** **fennel oil** **ginkgo** **St. John's wort** **wormwood**	May reduce seizure threshold and increase risk of seizures.	▪ Discourage use together, especially if pt has history of seizures. ▪ Monitor pt for seizure activity.
kava	May hinder therapy with CNS stimulants.	▪ Advise pt of this effect. ▪ Monitor pt for clinical effect.
sage	May induce seizures.	▪ Discourage use together.

Herb	Possible effects	Clinical tips
methylphenidate *(continued)*		
yohimbe bark	Potentiates hypertensive effects.	▪ Advise pt of this effect. ▪ Monitor BP.
methylprednisolone • Depo-Medrol, Depo-Predate, Medrol, Solu-Medrol		
alfalfa astragalus echinacea European mistletoe melatonin	May interfere with immunosuppressive effect of drug.	▪ Advise pt of this effect. ▪ Discourage use together. ▪ Watch for loss of therapeutic effect of drug.
aloe buckthorn cascara sagrada ephedra senna	May increase potassium loss.	▪ Monitor pt for signs and symptoms of hypokalemia, including muscle weakness, fatigue, nausea, vomiting, constipation, respiratory depression, and arrhythmias.
licorice	May interfere with immunosuppressive effect of drug or may increase drug plasma levels and potentiate its effects.	▪ Monitor pt for loss of therapeutic effectiveness of drug or signs and symptoms of corticosteroid toxicity.
metoclopramide hydrochloride • Apo-Metoclop ♦, Clopra, Maxeran ♦, Reclomide, Reglan		
borage **evening primrose oil** **fennel oil** **ginkgo**	May reduce seizure threshold.	▪ Discourage use together. ▪ Monitor pt for seizures.

Herb	Effect	Intervention
St. John's wort **wormwood**		
capsicum catnip goldenseal **kava** lady's slipper lemon balm melatonin nettle passion flower sassafras skullcap valerian	May cause excessive physical depression, sedation, and impairment. Use of kava may cause coma.	▪ Discourage use together. ▪ Monitor pt for signs and symptoms of increased CNS depression, including sedation, dizziness, ataxia, altered mental status, and respiratory depression.
ginger	May decrease nausea caused by chemo.	▪ May be used for increased therapeutic effect.
metoprolol • Apo-Metoprolol ◆, Betaloc ◆, Lopresor ◆, Lopresor SR ◆, Lopressor, Novo-Metoprol ◆, Nu-Metop ◆, Toprol-XL		
black cohosh *Coleus forskohlii*	May relax blood vessels and have unpredictable effects on BP if combined with beta blockers.	▪ Advise pt of this effect. ▪ Monitor BP closely.
ephedra	May increase BP because of unopposed sympathetic stimulation.	▪ Monitor pt for changes in BP and heart rate, arrhythmias, and shortness of breath.
goldenseal yohimbe bark	May interfere with drug's action because of herb's hypertensive properties.	▪ Advise pt of this effect. ▪ Monitor BP.
licorice	May increase sodium, chloride, and H_2O retention, resulting in BP increase.	▪ Monitor BP.

Herb	Possible effects	Clinical tips
metoprolol *(continued)*		
lily-of-the-valley	May increase risk of bradycardia or heart block.	▪ Monitor vital signs and ECG closely.
metronidazole • Apo-Metronidazole ♦, Flagyl, Flagyl ER, Novo-Nidazol ♦, Protostat, Trikacide ♦		
borage **evening primrose oil** **fennel oil** **ginkgo** **St. John's wort** **wormwood**	May reduce seizure threshold and increase risk of seizures.	▪ Discourage use together. ▪ Monitor pt for seizure activity.
mezlocillin sodium • Mezlin		
aloe buckthorn cascara sagrada Chinese rhubarb frangula guarana licorice senna	May decrease potassium level because of hypokalemia caused by use of herb.	▪ Monitor potassium level. ▪ Monitor pt for signs and symptoms of hypokalemia, including muscle weakness, fatigue, nausea, vomiting, constipation, respiratory depression, and arrhythmias.
bitter melon **fenugreek** **skullcap** **woundwort**	May cause hepatotoxicity.	▪ Monitor LFT values. ▪ Signs and symptoms of liver damage include abdominal pain, fever, malaise, jaundice, dark urine, clay-colored stools, and increased LFT values.

Herb	Effect	Nursing considerations
boneset **butterbur** **chaparral** **coltsfoot** **comfrey**	Contains pyrrolizidine alkaloids, which may be hepatotoxic.	▪ Signs and symptoms of liver damage include abdominal pain, fever, malaise, jaundice, dark urine, clay-colored stools, and increased LFT values.
echinacea	May increase hepatotoxicity if used with drugs that elevate liver enzyme levels.	▪ Advise pt of this adverse effect. ▪ Monitor LFT values.
khat	May decrease drug's antimicrobial effect.	▪ Advise pt to avoid herb for at least 2 h after taking drug.
midazolam hydrochloride • Versed, Versed Syrup		
capsicum catnip goldenseal **kava** lady's slipper lemon balm melatonin nettle passion flower sassafras skullcap valerian	May cause excessive physical depression, sedation, and impairment. Use of kava may cause coma.	▪ Discourage use together. ▪ Monitor pt for signs and symptoms of increased CNS depression, including sedation, dizziness, ataxia, altered mental status, and respiratory depression.
linden	May increase side effects of benzodiazepines because herb contains similar components.	▪ Advise pt to avoid excessive amounts of herb.

Herb	Possible effects	Clinical tips
miglitol • Glyset		
aloe bilberry leaf bitter melon bladderwrack burdock dandelion fenugreek garlic ginseng goat's rue gymnema	May improve glucose control, requiring a reduction of antidiabetics. May stimulate endogenous insulin release.	▪ Advise pt to consult health care provider before using herb. ▪ Monitor glucose level. ▪ Monitor pt for signs and symptoms of hypoglycemia, such as dizziness, diaphoresis, confusion, and tachycardia.
angelica broom buchu juniper ma huang	May decrease drug's hypoglycemic effect because of herbs' hyperglycemic properties.	▪ Monitor glucose level. ▪ Monitor pt for signs and symptoms of hyperglycemia (fatigue, polyuria, altered mental status, glucosuria, and ketonuria).
basil bay bee pollen burdock ginkgo biloba ginseng glucomannan horehound marshmallow	May affect glycemic control or disrupt a previously stable medical regimen.	▪ Monitor glucose level. ▪ Monitor pt for signs and symptoms of hyperglycemia (fatigue, polyuria, polydipsia, wt loss, abdominal pain, altered mental status, tachycardia, hypotension, glucosuria, ketonuria) or hypoglycemia (dizziness, diaphoresis, confusion, tachycardia). ▪ Dosage adjustments may be needed.

Herb	Effect	Nursing considerations
myrrh sage senega root yarrow		
fumitory **gossypol** **juniper** **oak bark** **wild ginger** **wintergreen** **yohimbe**	May increase risk of nephrotoxicity or RF.	▪ Reduced renal function may increase risk of hypoglycemia because of decreased drug elimination. ▪ Monitor results of renal function studies. ▪ Monitor pt for hypoglycemia.
modafinil • Provigil		
bitter melon **fenugreek** **skullcap** **woundwort** **yerba maté**	May cause hepatotoxicity.	▪ Monitor LFT values. ▪ Signs and symptoms of liver damage include abdominal pain, fever, malaise, jaundice, dark urine, clay-colored stools, and increased LFT values.
boldo	Stimulates the CNS, causing exaggerated reflexes, incoordination, and seizures.	▪ Discourage use together. ▪ Watch for CNS overstimulation.
cacao tree cola ephedra ginseng green tea guarana	May increase CNS stimulation.	▪ Advise pt of this effect and discourage use together. ▪ Monitor pt for increased stimulant effects, such as insomnia, irritability, dizziness, HTN, tachycardia, and palpitations.

Herb	Possible effects	Clinical tips
modafinil *(continued)*		
yerba maté yohimbe	May increase CNS stimulation.	▪ Advise pt of this effect and discourage use together. ▪ Monitor pt for increased stimulant effects, such as insomnia, irritability, dizziness, HTN, tachycardia, and palpitations.
kava	May hinder therapy with CNS stimulants.	▪ Advise pt of this effect. ▪ Monitor pt for clinical effect.
yohimbe bark	Potentiates hypertensive effects.	▪ Advise pt of this effect and monitor BP.
morphine hydrochloride, morphine sulfate • Astramorph PF, Duramorph, Epimorph ♦, Infumorph, Infumorph 500, Morphine H.P. ♦, Morphitec ♦, M.O.S. ♦, M.O.S.-S.R. ♦, MS Contin, MSIR, MS/L, Oramorph SR, RMS Uniserts, Roxanol, Statex		
bitter melon **fenugreek** **skullcap** **woundwort** **yerba maté**	May cause hepatotoxicity. Hepatic dysfunction may prolong drug effects.	▪ Discourage use together. ▪ Monitor LFT values. ▪ Signs and symptoms of liver damage include abdominal pain, fever, malaise, jaundice, dark urine, clay-colored stools.
boneset **butterbur** **chaparral** **coltsfoot** **comfrey**	Contains pyrrolizidine alkaloids, which may be hepatotoxic. Hepatic dysfunction may prolong drug effects.	▪ Discourage use together. ▪ Signs and symptoms of liver damage include abdominal pain, fever, malaise, jaundice, dark urine, clay-colored stools, and increased LFT values.
capsicum catnip goldenseal **kava** lady's slipper	May cause excessive physical depression, sedation, and impairment. Use of kava may cause coma.	▪ Discourage use together. ▪ Monitor pt for signs and symptoms of increased CNS depression, including sedation, dizziness, ataxia, altered mental status, and respiratory depression.

lemon balm melatonin nettle passion flower sassafras skullcap valerian		
fumitory **gossypol** **juniper** **oak bark** **wild ginger** **wintergreen** **yohimbe**	May increase risk of nephrotoxicity or RF. Renal dysfunction may prolong drug effects.	▪ Inform pt of the nephrotoxic potential of these herbs. ▪ Monitor results of renal function studies. ▪ Discourage use together.
oak bark	May reduce absorption of drug.	▪ Monitor pt for clinical effect.
snakeroot	May increase risk of renal problems because one component of snakeroot, aristolochic acid, has nephrotoxic properties.	▪ Discourage use together because of herb's toxic and carcinogenic potential.

moxifloxacin • Avelox

borage **evening primrose oil** **fennel oil** **ginkgo** **St. John's wort** **wormwood**	May reduce seizure threshold, increasing risk of seizures.	▪ Discourage use together. ▪ Monitor pt for seizure activity.

Herb	Possible effects	Clinical tips
moxifloxacin *(continued)*		
echinacea	May increase hepatotoxicity if used with drugs that elevate liver enzyme levels.	▪ Advise pt of this adverse effect. ▪ Monitor LFT values.
fennel	May reduce blood levels of ciprofloxacin, possibly impairing drug's effectiveness; may interfere similarly with other fluoroquinolone antibiotics.	▪ Discourage use together. ▪ Advise pt to separate times of use by 2 h to reduce the potential for an interaction.
nadolol • Corgard		
black cohosh *Coleus forskohlii*	Relaxes blood vessels and may have unpredictable effects on BP if combined with beta blockers.	▪ Advise pt of this effect. ▪ Monitor BP closely.
ephedra	May increase BP because of unopposed sympathetic stimulation.	▪ Monitor pt for changes in BP and heart rate, arrhythmias, and shortness of breath.
goldenseal yohimbe bark	May interfere with the drug's action because these herbs have hypertensive properties.	▪ Advise pt of this effect. ▪ Monitor BP.
licorice	May increase sodium, chloride, and H_2O retention, resulting in BP increase.	▪ Monitor BP.
lily-of-the-valley	May increase risk of bradycardia or heart block.	▪ Monitor vital signs and ECG closely.
nafcillin • Nallpen, Unipen		
khat	May decrease the antimicrobial effect of drug.	▪ Discourage use of herb for at least 2 h after taking drug.

naproxen • Apo-Naproxen ♦, EC-Naprosyn, Naprosyn, Naprosyn-E ♦, Naprosyn-SR, Naxen ♦, Novo-Naprox ♦, Nu-Naprox ♦		
agrimony bitter orange celery seed coriander dong quai fennel khella lovage motherwort Queen Anne's lace rosemary (topical) St. John's wort	May increase photosensitivity, adding to risk of sunburn or rash.	▪ Advise pt to wear a sunscreen or protective clothing during sun exposure.
angelica root anise bilberry borage seed oil danshen devil's claw dong quai echinacea feverfew garlic ginger ginkgo biloba	May increase risk of bleeding because of coumarin or coumarin derivatives in the herb or because of the herb's antiplatelet activity.	▪ Advise pt to consult health care provider before using herb. ▪ Monitor pt for signs of increased bleeding, including bruising, petechiae, bleeding gums, epistaxis, prolonged bleeding, melena, GI bleeding, hematuria, and hematemesis. ▪ Monitor results of hematologic and coagulation studies.

Herb	Possible effects	Clinical tips
naproxen *(continued)*		
horse chestnut licorice passion flower red clover	May increase risk of bleeding because of coumarin or coumarin derivatives in the herb or because of the herb's antiplatelet activity.	▪ Advise pt to consult health care provider before using herb. ▪ Monitor pt for signs of increased bleeding, including bruising, petechiae, bleeding gums, epistaxis, prolonged bleeding, melena, GI bleeding, hematuria, and hematemesis. ▪ Monitor results of hematologic and coagulation studies.
bitter melon **fenugreek** **skullcap** **woundwort** **yerba maté**	May cause hepatotoxicity.	▪ Monitor LFT values. ▪ Signs and symptoms of liver damage include abdominal pain, fever, malaise, jaundice, dark urine, clay-colored stools, and increased LFT values.
boneset **butterbur** **chaparral** **coltsfoot** **comfrey**	Contains pyrrolizidine alkaloids, which may be hepatotoxic.	▪ Discourage use. ▪ Signs and symptoms of liver damage include abdominal pain, fever, malaise, jaundice, dark urine, clay-colored stools, and increased LFT values.
capsicum	Stimulates GI secretions to help protect against NSAID-induced GI irritation.	▪ May be used for therapeutic advantage.
Coffea arabica cola gossypol uva-ursi	May cause increased adverse GI effects.	▪ Advise pt of increased risk of adverse GI effects.
echinacea	May increase hepatotoxicity.	▪ Advise pt of this adverse effect. Monitor LFT values.

fumitory **gossypol** **juniper** **oak bark** **wild ginger** **wintergreen** **yohimbe**	May increase risk of nephrotoxicity or RF.	▪ Pt may be unaware of the nephrotoxic potential of these herbs. ▪ Monitor results of renal function studies.
kava	May increase risk of hepatic adverse reactions, such as cirrhosis, hepatitis, or liver failure.	▪ Discourage use together. ▪ Monitor LFT values. ▪ Advise pt to report signs and symptoms of liver problems to health care provider.
meadowsweet white willow	May increase risk of bleeding because of salicylates in the herb.	▪ Monitor pt for signs and symptoms of increased bleeding, including bruising, petechiae, bleeding gums, epistaxis, prolonged bleeding after injury, melena, GI bleeding, hematuria, and hematemesis. ▪ Monitor results of hematologic studies and coagulation studies.
nefazodone • Serzone		
capsicum catnip goldenseal **kava** lady's slipper lemon balm melatonin nettle	May cause excessive physical depression, sedation, and impairment. Use of kava may cause coma.	▪ Discourage use together. ▪ Monitor pt for signs and symptoms of increased CNS depression, including sedation, dizziness, ataxia, altered mental status, and respiratory depression.

Herb	Possible effects	Clinical tips
nefazodone *(continued)*		
passion flower sassafras skullcap valerian	May cause excessive physical depression, sedation, and impairment.	▪ Discourage use together. ▪ Monitor pt for signs and symptoms of increased CNS depression, including sedation, dizziness, ataxia, altered mental status, and respiratory depression.
St. John's wort	May cause excitation, hyperpyrexia, seizures, delirium, or coma.	▪ Discourage use together.
nelfinavir • Viracept		
bitter melon **fenugreek** **skullcap** **woundwort** **yerba maté**	May cause hepatotoxicity.	▪ Monitor LFT values. ▪ Signs and symptoms of liver damage include abdominal pain, fever, malaise, jaundice, dark urine, clay-colored stools, and increased LFT values.
boneset **butterbur** **chaparral** **coltsfoot** **comfrey**	Contains pyrrolizidine alkaloids, which may be hepatotoxic.	▪ Discourage use together. ▪ Signs and symptoms of liver damage include abdominal pain, fever, malaise, jaundice, dark urine, clay-colored stools, and increased LFT values.
echinacea	May increase hepatotoxicity if used with drugs that elevate liver enzyme levels. May exacerbate HIV infect or AIDS.	▪ Advise pt of these effects. ▪ Discourage use together.
garlic	Use with protease inhibitors may cause severe GI toxicity.	▪ Discourage use together.

Herb	Effect	Nursing considerations
	May reduce the effectiveness of some drugs used for HIV.	
St. John's wort	Reduces indinavir levels by more than 50%; may have similar effects with other protease inhibitors.	▪ Discourage use together.
nevirapine • Viramune		
bitter melon **fenugreek** **skullcap** **woundwort** **yerba maté**	May cause hepatotoxicity.	▪ Monitor LFT values. ▪ Signs and symptoms of liver damage include abdominal pain, fever, malaise, jaundice, dark urine, clay-colored stools, and increased LFT values.
boneset **butterbur** **chaparral** **coltsfoot** **comfrey**	Contains pyrrolizidine alkaloids, which may be hepatotoxic.	▪ Discourage use together. ▪ Signs and symptoms of liver damage include abdominal pain, fever, malaise, jaundice, dark urine, clay-colored stools, and increased LFT values.
echinacea	May increase hepatotoxicity if used with drugs that elevate liver enzyme levels. May exacerbate HIV infect or AIDS.	▪ Discourage use together in pt taking antiviral.
kava	May increase risk of hepatic adverse reactions, such as cirrhosis, hepatitis, or liver failure.	▪ Discourage use together. ▪ Monitor LFT values. ▪ Advise pt to report signs and symptoms of liver problems to health care provider.
St. John's wort	Induces the cytochrome P450 metabolic pathway, which may decrease therapeutic	▪ Advise pt to avoid use. Pt should consult health care provider before using herbs.

(continued)

Herb	Possible effects	Clinical tips
nevirapine *(continued)*		
St. John's wort *(continued)*	effects of drugs that use this pathway for metabolism. May cause subtherapeutic antiretroviral levels and insufficient virologic response, leading to resistance or class cross-resistance.	
nifedipine • Adalat, Adalat CC, Adalat PA ◆, Adalat XL ◆, Apo-Nifed ◆, Novo-Nifedin ◆, Nu-Nifed ◆, Procardia, Procardia XL		
black cohosh	May increase peripheral vasodilation, resulting in hypotension.	▪ Monitor BP closely. ▪ Dosage adjustment may be needed.
cat's claw chicory	May increase antianginal effect.	▪ Advise pt to consult health care provider before taking herb.
ginger	May increase calcium uptake by the myocardium, leading to altered drug effects.	▪ Monitor pt for therapeutic effect. ▪ Discourage use together.
goldenseal yohimbe bark	May interfere with the drug's action because these herbs have hypertensive properties.	▪ Monitor pt for clinical effect. Monitor BP.
licorice	May increase sodium, chloride, and H_2O retention, resulting in BP increase.	▪ Monitor BP.
lily-of-the-valley	May increase risk of bradycardia or heart block.	▪ Monitor vital signs and ECG closely.
nitrofurantoin macrocrystals • Macrobid, Macrodantin		
bitter melon	May cause hepatotoxicity.	▪ Monitor LFT values.

fenugreek **skullcap** **woundwort** **yerba maté**		▪ Signs and symptoms of liver damage include abdominal pain, fever, malaise, jaundice, dark urine, clay-colored stools, and increased LFT values.
boneset **butterbur** **chaparral** **coltsfoot** **comfrey**	Contains pyrrolizidine alkaloids, which may be hepatotoxic.	▪ Signs and symptoms of liver damage include abdominal pain, fever, malaise, jaundice, dark urine, clay-colored stools, and increased LFT values.
echinacea	May increase hepatotoxicity if used with drugs that elevate liver enzyme levels.	▪ Advise pt of this adverse effect. ▪ Monitor LFT values.
fumitory **gossypol** **juniper** **oak bark** **wild ginger** **wintergreen** **yohimbe**	May increase risk of nephrotoxicity or RF. Renal impairment increases risk of drug toxicity, particularly peripheral neuropathy.	▪ Inform pt of herb's nephrotoxic potential. ▪ Monitor results of renal function studies.
kava	May increase risk of hepatic adverse reactions, such as cirrhosis, hepatitis, or liver failure.	▪ Discourage use together. ▪ Monitor LFT values. ▪ Advise pt to report signs and symptoms of liver problems to health care provider.
snakeroot	May increase risk of renal problems because one component of snakeroot, aristolochic acid, has nephrotoxic properties.	▪ Discourage use together because of herb's toxic and carcinogenic potential.

Herb	Possible effects	Clinical tips
nortriptyline • Aventyl, Pamelor		
agrimony bitter orange celery seed coriander dong quai fennel khella lovage motherwort Queen Anne's lace rosemary (topical) St. John's wort	May increase photosensitivity, adding to risk of sunburn or rash.	▪ Advise pt to wear a sunscreen or protective clothing during sun exposure.
borage **evening primrose oil** **fennel oil** **ginkgo** **St. John's wort** **wormwood**	May reduce seizure threshold, increasing risk of seizures.	▪ Discourage use together, especially if pt has seizure history. ▪ Monitor pt for seizure activity.
capsicum ephedra Scotch broom yohimbe	May cause HTN in pt taking TCA.	▪ Discourage use together. ▪ Monitor BP.

capsicum catnip goldenseal **kava** lady's slipper lemon balm melatonin nettle passion flower sassafras skullcap valerian	May cause excessive physical depression, sedation, and impairment. Use of kava may cause coma.	▪ Discourage use together. ▪ Monitor pt for signs and symptoms of increased CNS depression, including sedation, dizziness, ataxia, altered mental status, and respiratory depression.
sage	May induce seizures.	▪ Discourage use together.
SAMe **St. John's wort** **yohimbe**	May cause elevation of serotonin levels.	▪ Discourage use together. ▪ Monitor pt for signs and symptoms of serotonin syn, including nausea, hypotension, HTN, excitation, mental status changes, hyperpyrexia, and coma.
St. John's wort	May cause decreased tricyclic plasma levels, resulting in decreased therapeutic effects.	▪ Discourage use together. ▪ Monitor pt for adequate therapeutic response.
ofloxacin • Floxin, Floxin I.V.		
agrimony bitter orange celery seed coriander dong quai	May increase photosensitivity, adding to risk of sunburn or rash.	▪ Advise pt to wear a sunscreen or protective clothing during sun exposure.

Herb	Possible effects	Clinical tips
ofloxacin *(continued)*		
fennel khella lovage motherwort Queen Anne's lace rosemary (topical) St. John's wort	May increase photosensitivity, adding to risk of sunburn or rash.	▪ Advise pt to wear a sunscreen or protective clothing during sun exposure.
borage **evening primrose oil** **fennel oil** **ginkgo** **St. John's wort** **wormwood**	May reduce seizure threshold, increasing risk of seizures.	▪ Discourage use together because such use may lower seizure threshold. ▪ Monitor pt for seizure activity.
echinacea	May increase hepatotoxicity.	▪ Advise pt of this adverse effect. ▪ Monitor LFT values.
fennel	May reduce drug levels, possibly impairing its effectiveness.	▪ Advise pt to separate use by 2 h to reduce the potential for an interaction. ▪ Discourage use together.
fumitory **gossypol**	May increase risk of nephrotoxicity or RF.	▪ Inform pt of herb's nephrotoxic potential. ▪ Monitor results of renal function studies.

...r **...k** **...ger** **...intergreen** **yohimbe**		
kava	May increase risk of hepatic adverse reactions, such as cirrhosis, hepatitis, or liver failure.	▪ Discourage use together. ▪ Monitor LFT values. ▪ Advise pt to report signs and symptoms of liver problems to health care provider.
snakeroot	May increase risk of renal problems because one component of snakeroot, aristolochic acid, has nephrotoxic properties.	▪ Discourage use together because of herb's toxic and carcinogenic potential.
olanzapine • Zyprexa		
borage **evening primrose oil** **fennel oil** **ginkgo** **St. John's wort** **wormwood**	May reduce seizure threshold, increasing risk of seizures.	▪ Discourage use together, especially if pt has seizure history. ▪ Monitor pt for seizure activity.
capsicum catnip goldenseal **kava** lady's slipper lemon balm	May cause excessive physical depression, sedation, and impairment. Use of kava may cause coma.	▪ Discourage use together. ▪ Monitor pt for signs and symptoms of increased CNS depression, including sedation, dizziness, ataxia, altered mental status, and respiratory depression.

Herb	Possible effects	Clinical tips
olanzapine *(continued)*		
melatonin nettle passion flower sassafras skullcap valerian	May cause excessive physical depression, sedation, and impairment.	▪ Discourage use together. ▪ Monitor pt for signs and symptoms of increased CNS depression, including sedation, dizziness, ataxia, altered mental status, and respiratory depression.
ginseng ma huang	Herb may act as CNS stimulant.	▪ Discourage use together. ▪ Avoid use with antipsychotics.
nutmeg	May cause a loss of symptom control or interfere with existing therapy for psychiatric illnesses.	▪ Discourage use together. ▪ Monitor pt for clinical effect.
sage	May induce seizures.	▪ Discourage use together.
St. John's wort	May reduce drug levels, increasing severity of psychotic symptoms. If drug levels are adjusted for pt taking St. John's wort, stopping the herb could cause these levels to rise, potentially causing toxicity.	▪ Discourage use together. ▪ Monitor pt for clinical effect. ▪ Dosage adjustment may be needed if St. John's wort is discontinued during drug therapy.
omeprazole • Losec ♦, Prilosec		
agrimony bitter orange celery seed coriander dong quai	May increase photosensitivity, adding to risk of sunburn or rash.	▪ Advise pt to wear a sunscreen or protective clothing during sun exposure.

Herb	Effect	Action
fennel khella lovage motherwort Queen Anne's lace rosemary (topical) St. John's wort		
blessed thistle bogbean capsicum ginger goldenseal mustard sweet flag true unicorn root yarrow yew	May decrease drug effect because herb causes increased acid secretion.	▪ Advise pt of this effect. ▪ Monitor pt for clinical effect.
male fern	Alkaline environment deactivates herb.	▪ Advise pt of this effect.
pennyroyal	May change rate of formation of toxic metabolites of pennyroyal.	▪ Advise pt of this effect. ▪ Discourage use unless approved by health care provider.
ondansetron hydrochloride • Zofran		
bitter melon **fenugreek**	May cause hepatotoxicity.	▪ Monitor LFT values. ▪ Signs and symptoms of liver damage

(continued)

Herb	Possible effects	Clinical tips
ondansetron hydrochloride *(continued)*		
skullcap **woundwort** **yerba maté**		include abdominal pain, fever, malaise, jaundice, dark urine, clay-colored stools, and increased LFT values.
boneset **butterbur** **chaparral** **coltsfoot** **comfrey**	Contains pyrrolizidine alkaloids, which may be hepatotoxic.	▪ Signs and symptoms of liver damage include abdominal pain, fever, malaise, jaundice, dark urine, clay-colored stools, and increased LFT values.
echinacea	May increase hepatotoxicity if used with drugs that elevate liver enzyme levels.	▪ Advise pt of this adverse effect. ▪ Monitor LFT values.
ginger	May decrease nausea caused by chemo.	▪ May be used for therapeutic effect.
kava	May increase risk of hepatic adverse reactions, such as cirrhosis, hepatitis, or liver failure.	▪ Discourage use together. ▪ Monitor LFT values. ▪ Advise pt to report signs and symptoms of liver problems to health care provider.
oxazepam • Apo-Oxazepam ◆, Novoxapam ◆, Serax		
capsicum catnip goldenseal **kava** lady's slipper lemon balm melatonin	May cause excessive physical depression, sedation, and impairment. Use of kava may cause coma.	▪ Discourage use together. ▪ Monitor pt for signs and symptoms of increased CNS depression, including sedation, dizziness, ataxia, altered mental status, and respiratory depression.

Herb	Interaction	Nursing considerations
nettle passion flower sassafras skullcap valerian		
linden	May increase adverse effects of benzodiazepine because herb contains similar components.	▪ Advise pt to avoid excessive amounts of herb.
yohimbe	May block action of drug.	▪ Monitor pt for clinical effect.
oxcarbazepine • Trileptal		
borage **evening primrose oil** **fennel oil** **ginkgo** **St. John's wort** **wormwood**	May decrease effectiveness of anticonvulsants; may reduce seizure threshold.	▪ Discourage use together.
capsicum catnip goldenseal **kava** lady's slipper lemon balm melatonin nettle passion flower	May cause excessive physical depression, sedation, and impairment. Use of kava may cause coma.	▪ Discourage use together. ▪ Monitor pt for signs of increased CNS depression, including sedation, ataxia, altered mental status, and respiratory depression.

Herb	Possible effects	Clinical tips
oxcarbazepine *(continued)*		
sassafras skullcap valerian	May cause excessive physical depression, sedation, and impairment.	▪ Discourage use together. ▪ Monitor pt for signs of increased CNS depression, including sedation, ataxia, altered mental status, and respiratory depression.
hyssop	May counteract the antiseizure effects of anticonvulsants.	▪ Advise pt of this effect. ▪ Advise pt to consult health care provider before using herb.
nettle	May increase sedative adverse effects. May increase risk of seizures.	▪ Discourage use together.
sage	May induce seizures.	▪ Advise pt to consult health care provider before using herb.
paclitaxel • Taxol		
bitter melon **fenugreek** **skullcap** **woundwort** **yerba maté**	May cause hepatotoxicity.	▪ Monitor LFT values. ▪ Signs and symptoms of liver damage include abdominal pain, fever, malaise, jaundice, dark urine, clay-colored stools, and increased LFT values.
boneset **butterbur** **chaparral** **coltsfoot** **comfrey**	Contains pyrrolizidine alkaloids, which may be hepatotoxic.	▪ Signs and symptoms of liver damage include abdominal pain, fever, malaise, jaundice, dark urine, clay-colored stools, and increased LFT values.
echinacea	May increase hepatotoxicity if used with drugs that elevate liver enzyme levels.	▪ Advise pt of this adverse effect. ▪ Monitor LFT values.

ginger	May decrease nausea caused by chemo.	▪ May be used for clinical effect.
kava	May increase risk of hepatic adverse reactions, such as cirrhosis, hepatitis, or liver failure.	▪ Discourage use together. ▪ Monitor LFT values. ▪ Advise pt to report signs and symptoms of liver problems to health care provider.
yew	May potentiate myelosuppression and interactions with other chemo drugs.	▪ Monitor results of hematologic studies. ▪ Monitor pt for increased adverse effects. ▪ Discourage use of herbs unless approved by health care provider.
pantoprazole • Protonix		
bitter melon **fenugreek** **skullcap** **woundwort** **yerba maté**	May cause hepatotoxicity.	▪ Monitor LFT values. ▪ Signs and symptoms of liver damage include abdominal pain, fever, malaise, jaundice, dark urine, clay-colored stools, and increased LFT values.
blessed thistle bogbean capsicum ginger goldenseal mustard sweet flag true unicorn root yarrow yew	May decrease drug effectiveness because herbs cause increased acid secretion.	▪ Advise pt of this effect. ▪ Monitor pt for clinical effect.

Herb	Possible effects	Clinical tips
pantoprazole *(continued)*		
boneset **butterbur** **chaparral** **coltsfoot** **comfrey**	Contains pyrrolizidine alkaloids, which may be hepatotoxic.	▪ Signs and symptoms of liver damage include abdominal pain, fever, malaise, jaundice, dark urine, clay-colored stools, and increased LFT values.
echinacea	May increase hepatotoxicity.	▪ Advise pt of this effect. ▪ Monitor LFT values.
paroxetine • Paxil, Paxil CR		
5-HTP	May cause serotonin syn.	▪ Discourage use together. ▪ Monitor pt for symptoms, including nausea, hypotension, HTN, excitation, mental status changes, hyperpyrexia, and coma.
ginkgo	May reduce the sexual adverse effects of SSRIs in both men and women.	▪ Advise pt of this effect.
St. John's wort	May cause serotonin syn.	▪ Discourage use together. ▪ Advise pt switching from SSRI to St. John's wort to wait a few weeks for the SSRI to wash out of his system before it's safe to start taking the herb. The exact time required depends on which SSRI was used. ▪ Advise pt to consult health care provider before using herb.
SAMe	May increase dopamine levels.	▪ Discourage use together.
yohimbe	May cause serotonin syn.	▪ Discourage use together.

penicillin		
fumitory **gossypol** **juniper** **oak bark** **wild ginger** **wintergreen** **yohimbe**	May increase risk of nephrotoxicity or RF. May increase risk of renal damage when combined with drug.	▪ Inform pt of herb's nephrotoxic potential. ▪ Monitor results of renal function studies.
khat	May decrease antimicrobial effect of drug.	▪ Advise pt to avoid herb for at least 2 h after taking drug.
snakeroot	May increase risk of renal problems because one component of snakeroot, aristolochic acid, has nephrotoxic properties.	▪ Discourage use together because of herb's toxic and carcinogenic potential.

phenytoin sodium (extended) • Dilantin Kapseals		
agrimony bitter orange celery seed coriander dong quai fennel khella lovage motherwort Queen Anne's lace	May increase photosensitivity, adding to risk of sunburn or rash.	▪ Advise pt to wear a sunscreen and protective clothing during sun exposure.

Herb	Possible effects	Clinical tips
phenytoin sodium (extended) *(continued)*		
rosemary (topical) St. John's wort	May increase photosensitivity, adding to risk of sunburn or rash.	▪ Advise pt to wear a sunscreen and protective clothing during sun exposure.
bitter melon **fenugreek** **skullcap** **woundwort** **yerba maté**	May cause hepatotoxicity.	▪ Monitor LFT values. ▪ Signs and symptoms of liver damage include abdominal pain, fever, malaise, jaundice, dark urine, clay-colored stools, and increased LFT values.
boneset **butterbur** **chaparral** **coltsfoot** **comfrey**	Contains pyrrolizidine alkaloids, which may be hepatotoxic.	▪ Signs and symptoms of liver damage include abdominal pain, fever, malaise, jaundice, dark urine, clay-colored stools, and increased LFT values.
borage **evening primrose oil** **fennel oil** **ginkgo** **St. John's wort** **wormwood**	May decrease effectiveness of anticonvulsants. May reduce seizure threshold.	▪ Discourage use together.
echinacea	May increase hepatotoxicity if used with drugs that elevate liver enzyme levels.	▪ Advise pt of this adverse effect. ▪ Monitor LFT values.

Herb	Effect	Nursing considerations
hyssop	May counteract antiseizure effects of anticonvulsants.	▪ Advise pt of this effect. ▪ Advise pt to consult health care provider before using herbs.
nettle	May increase sedative adverse effects. May increase risk of seizures.	▪ Discourage use together.
sage	May induce seizures.	▪ Advise pt to consult health care provider before using herbs.
pioglitazone • Actos		
aloe bilberry leaf bitter melon bladderwrack burdock dandelion fenugreek garlic ginseng goat's rue gymnema	May improve glucose control, requiring a reduction of antidiabetic. May stimulate endogenous insulin release.	▪ Advise pt to consult health care provider before using herbs. ▪ Monitor glucose level. ▪ Monitor pt for signs and symptoms of hypoglycemia, such as dizziness, diaphoresis, confusion, and tachycardia.
angelica broom buchu juniper ma huang	May decrease drug's hypoglycemic effect because of herb's hyperglycemic properties.	▪ Monitor glucose level. ▪ Monitor pt for signs and symptoms of hyperglycemia (fatigue, polyuria, altered mental status, glucosuria, and ketonuria).
basil bay bee pollen	May affect glycemic control and disrupt a previously stable medical regimen.	▪ Monitor glucose level. ▪ Monitor pt for signs and symptoms of hyperglycemia (fatigue, polyuria, polydipsia, wt loss, abdominal *(continued)*

Herb	Possible effects	Clinical tips
pioglitazone *(continued)*		
burdock ginkgo biloba ginseng glucomannan horehound marshmallow myrrh sage senega root yarrow		pain, altered mental status, tachycardia, hypotension, glucosuria, ketonuria) or hypoglycemia (dizziness, diaphoresis, confusion, tachycardia). ▪ Dosage adjustments may be needed.
bitter melon **fenugreek** **skullcap** **woundwort** **yerba maté**	May cause hepatotoxicity.	▪ May cause hepatotoxicity. ▪ Monitor LFT values. ▪ Signs and symptoms of liver damage include abdominal pain, fever, malaise, jaundice, dark urine, clay-colored stools, and increased LFT values.
boneset **butterbur** **chaparral** **coltsfoot** **comfrey**	Contains pyrrolizidine alkaloids, which may be hepatotoxic.	▪ May cause hepatotoxicity. ▪ Monitor LFT values. ▪ Signs and symptoms of liver damage include abdominal pain, fever, malaise, jaundice, dark urine, clay-colored stools, and increased LFT values.
piroxicam • Apo-Piroxicam ◆, Feldene, Novo-Pirocam ◆		
agrimony bitter orange celery seed	May increase photosensitivity, increasing risk of sunburn or skin rash.	▪ Advise pt to wear a sunscreen or protective clothing during sun exposure.

coriander dong quai fennel khella lovage motherwort Queen Anne's lace rosemary (topical) St. John's wort		
angelica root anise bilberry borage seed oil danshen devil's claw dong quai echinacea feverfew garlic ginger ginkgo biloba horse chestnut licorice passion flower red clover	May increase risk of bleeding because of coumarin or coumarin derivatives in the herb or because of the herb's antiplatelet activity.	▪ Monitor pt for signs and symptoms of increased bleeding, including bruising, petechiae, bleeding gums, epistaxis, prolonged bleeding after injury, melena, GI bleeding, hematuria, and hematemesis. ▪ Monitor results of hematologic studies and coagulation studies. ▪ Advise pt to consult health care provider before using herb.

Herb	Possible effects	Clinical tips
piroxicam *(continued)*		
bitter melon **fenugreek** **skullcap** **woundwort** **yerba maté**	May cause hepatotoxicity.	▪ Monitor LFT values. ▪ Signs and symptoms of liver damage include abdominal pain, fever, malaise, jaundice, dark urine, clay-colored stools, and increased LFT values.
boneset **butterbur** **chaparral** **coltsfoot** **comfrey**	Contains pyrrolizidine alkaloids, which may be hepatotoxic.	▪ Discourage use together. ▪ Signs and symptoms of liver damage include abdominal pain, fever, malaise, jaundice, dark urine, clay-colored stools, and increased LFT values.
capsicum	Stimulates GI secretions to help protect against NSAID-induced GI irritation.	▪ May be used for therapeutic advantage.
Coffea arabica cola gossypol uva-ursi	May cause increased adverse GI effects.	▪ Advise pt of increased risk of adverse GI effects.
echinacea	May increase hepatotoxicity if used with drugs that elevate liver enzyme levels.	▪ Advise pt of this effect. ▪ Monitor LFT values.
fumitory **gossypol** **juniper** **oak bark** **wild ginger**	May increase risk of nephrotoxicity or RF.	▪ Pt may be unaware of the nephrotoxic potential of these herbs. ▪ Monitor results of renal function studies.

wintergreen **yohimbe**		
meadowsweet white willow	May increase risk of bleeding because of salicylates in the herb.	▪ Monitor pt for signs and symptoms of increased bleeding, including bruising, petechiae, bleeding gums, epistaxis, prolonged bleeding after injury, melena, GI bleeding, hematuria, and hematemesis. ▪ Monitor results of hematologic studies and coagulation studies.
snakeroot	May increase risk of renal problems because one component of snakeroot, aristolochic acid, has nephrotoxic properties.	▪ Discourage use together because of herb's toxic and carcinogenic potential.
wild yam	May decrease the anti-inflammatory effect of drug.	▪ Monitor pt for clinical effects.

pramipexole dihydrochloride • Mirapex

kava	May cause tremors, muscle spasms, or abnormal movements, decreasing the drug effect.	▪ Monitor pt for clinical effect. ▪ Discourage use together.
valerian	May increase CNS effects of the drug.	▪ Monitor pt for increased adverse effects.

pravastatin (eptastatin) • Pravachol

bitter melon **fenugreek** **skullcap** **woundwort** **yerba maté**	May cause hepatotoxicity.	▪ Monitor LFT values. Signs and symptoms of liver damage include abdominal pain, fever, malaise, jaundice, dark urine, clay-colored stools, and increased LFT values.

Herb	Possible effects	Clinical tips
pravastatin (eptastatin) *(continued)*		
boneset **butterbur** **chaparral** **coltsfoot** **comfrey**	Contains pyrrolizidine alkaloids, which may be hepatotoxic.	▪ Discourage use. Signs and symptoms of liver damage include abdominal pain, fever, malaise, jaundice, dark urine, clay-colored stools, and increased LFT values.
echinacea	May increase hepatotoxicity if used with drugs that elevate liver enzyme levels.	▪ Monitor LFT values.
garlic	May have additive lipid-lowering properties.	▪ May be used for therapeutic advantage.
pectin	May decrease the effectiveness of HMG-CoA reductase inhibitors.	▪ Discourage use together. Monitor pt for clinical response.
red yeast rice	Contains similar components to those of statin drugs, increasing risk of adverse events or toxicity.	▪ Discourage use together if possible. If these agents must be used together, monitor pt for signs and symptoms of increased adverse effects such as myopathy and rhabdomyolysis.
St. John's wort	May decrease blood levels of various drugs in the statin family.	▪ Monitor pt for clinical response.
prazosin hydrochloride • Minipress		
black cohosh	May increase peripheral vasodilation, resulting in hypotension.	▪ Monitor BP closely. ▪ Dosage adjustment may be needed.
butcher's broom	May reduce drug effects.	▪ Advise pt of this interaction. ▪ Monitor pt for clinical effect.
fenugreek	May increase vasodilatory effect.	▪ Monitor pt for increased hypotension.

goldenseal yohimbe bark	May interfere with the drug's action because these herbs have hypertensive properties.	▪ Monitor pt for clinical effect. ▪ Monitor BP.
licorice	May increase sodium, chloride, and H_2O retention, resulting in BP increase.	▪ Monitor BP.
saw palmetto	May increase alpha blocking effect when combined with alpha blockers.	▪ Monitor vital signs and ECG for adverse effects.
prednisone • Apo-Prednisone ◆, Deltasone, Liquid Pred, Meticorten, Orasone, Prednicen-M, Prednisone Intensol, Sterapred, Winpred ◆		
alfalfa astragalus echinacea European mistletoe melatonin	May interfere with immunosuppressive effect of drug.	▪ Advise pt of this effect. ▪ Discourage use together. ▪ Watch for loss of therapeutic effect of drug.
aloe buckthorn cascara sagrada ephedra senna	May increase potassium loss.	▪ Monitor pt for signs and symptoms of hypokalemia, including muscle weakness, fatigue, nausea, vomiting, constipation, respiratory depression, and arrhythmias.
licorice	May interfere with immunosuppressive effect of drug. May increase drug plasma levels. May potentiate drug effects.	▪ Monitor pt for loss of therapeutic effectiveness of drug and signs and symptoms of corticosteroid toxicity.

Herb	Possible effects	Clinical tips
prednisone *(continued)*		
morinda	May counteract the effects of immunosuppressants.	▪ Advise pt of this effect. ▪ Discourage use together. ▪ Watch for loss of therapeutic effect of drug.
prochlorperazine • Compazine, PMS Prochlorperazine ♦, Stemetil ♦		
agrimony bitter orange celery seed coriander dong quai fennel khella lovage motherwort Queen Anne's lace rosemary (topical) St. John's wort	May increase photosensitivity, adding to risk of sunburn or rash.	▪ Advise pt to wear a sunscreen or protective clothing during sun exposure.
bitter melon **fenugreek** **skullcap** **woundwort** **yerba maté**	May cause hepatotoxicity.	▪ Monitor LFT values. ▪ Signs and symptoms of liver damage include abdominal pain, fever, malaise, jaundice, dark urine, clay-colored stools, and increased LFT values.

boneset **butterbur** **chaparral** **coltsfoot** **comfrey**	Contains pyrrolizidine alkaloids, which may be hepatotoxic.	▪ Signs and symptoms of liver damage include abdominal pain, fever, malaise, jaundice, dark urine, clay-colored stools, and increased LFT values.
borage **evening primrose oil** **fennel oil** **ginkgo** **St. John's wort** **wormwood**	May reduce seizure threshold, increasing risk of seizures.	▪ Discourage use together, especially if pt has seizure history. ▪ Monitor pt for seizure activity.
butterbur corkwood henbane jimsonweed	Increases anticholinergic effects.	▪ Advise pt of this effect. ▪ Monitor pt for increased adverse effects, including headache, dizziness, confusion, irritability, tachycardia, mydriasis, dry mouth, constipation, urinary retention, and hot, dry skin.
capsicum catnip goldenseal **kava** lady's slipper lemon balm melatonin nettle passion flower sassafras	May cause excessive physical depression, sedation, and impairment. Use of kava may cause coma.	▪ Discourage use together. ▪ Monitor pt for signs of increased CNS depression, including sedation, ataxia, altered mental status, and respiratory depression.

Herb	Possible effects	Clinical tips
prochlorperazine *(continued)*		
skullcap valerian	May cause excessive physical depression, sedation, and impairment.	▪ Discourage use together. ▪ Monitor pt for signs of increased CNS depression, including sedation, ataxia, altered mental status, and respiratory depression.
echinacea	May increase hepatotoxicity if used with drugs that elevate liver enzyme levels.	▪ Advise pt of this adverse effect. ▪ Monitor LFT values.
ginseng ma huang	Herb may act as CNS stimulant.	▪ Discourage use together. ▪ Avoid use with antipsychotics.
nutmeg	May cause a loss of symptom control or interfere with existing therapy for psychiatric illnesses.	▪ Discourage use together. ▪ Monitor pt for clinical effect.
sage	May induce seizures.	▪ Discourage use together.
yohimbe	May increase risk of toxicity.	▪ Discourage use together. ▪ Monitor pt for adverse effects, including dizziness, psychoses, tachycardia, hypotension or HTN, GI complaints, and RF.
propoxyphene • Darvon-N, 642 ◆		
bitter melon **fenugreek** **skullcap** **woundwort** **yerba maté**	May cause hepatotoxicity. Hepatic dysfunction may prolong drug effects.	▪ Discourage use together. ▪ Monitor LFT values. ▪ Signs and symptoms of liver damage include abdominal pain, fever, malaise, jaundice, dark urine, clay-colored stools, and increased LFT values.
boneset	Contains pyrrolizidine alkaloids, which may	▪ Discourage use together.

butterbur **chaparral** **coltsfoot** **comfrey**	be hepatotoxic. Hepatic dysfunction may prolong drug effects.	▪ Signs and symptoms of liver damage include abdominal pain, fever, malaise, jaundice, dark urine, clay-colored stools, and increased LFT values.
capsicum catnip goldenseal **kava** lady's slipper lemon balm melatonin nettle passion flower sassafras skullcap valerian	May cause excessive physical depression, sedation, and impairment. Use of kava may cause coma.	▪ Discourage use together. ▪ Monitor pt for signs and symptoms of increased CNS depression, including sedation, dizziness, ataxia, altered mental status, and respiratory depression.
fumitory **gossypol** **juniper** **oak bark** **wild ginger** **wintergreen** **yohimbe**	May increase risk of nephrotoxicity or RF. Renal dysfunction may prolong drug effects.	▪ Inform pt of herb's nephrotoxic potential. ▪ Monitor results of renal function studies. ▪ Discourage use together.
snakeroot	May increase risk of renal problems because one component of snakeroot, aristolochic acid, has nephrotoxic properties.	▪ Discourage use together because of herb's toxic and carcinogenic potential.

Herb	Possible effects	Clinical tips
propranolol • Apo-Propranolol ◆, Inderal, Inderal LA, Novopranol ◆, pms Propranolol ◆		
black cohosh *Coleus forskohlii*	Relaxes blood vessels and may have unpredictable effects on BP if combined with beta blockers.	▪ Advise pt of this effect. ▪ Monitor BP closely.
ephedra	May increase BP because of unopposed sympathetic stimulation.	▪ Monitor pt for changes in BP and heart rate, arrhythmias, and shortness of breath.
goldenseal yohimbe bark	May interfere with the drug's action because these herbs have hypertensive properties.	▪ Advise pt of this effect. ▪ Monitor BP.
licorice	May increase sodium, chloride, and H_2O retention, resulting in BP increase.	▪ Monitor BP.
lily-of-the-valley	May increase risk of bradycardia or heart block.	▪ Monitor vital signs and ECG closely.
pseudoephedrine • Afrin, Allermed, Cenafed, Chlor-Trimeton Non-Drowsy Decongestant, Decofed, Drixoral Non-Drowsy Formula, Eltor 120 ◆, Halofed, Maxenal ◆, Novafed, Sinutab, Sudafed		
capsicum ma huang Scotch broom yohimbe	May cause increased sympathomimetic effects.	▪ Monitor pt for increased adverse effects.
ginseng	May potentiate CNS stimulant effects.	▪ Monitor pt for increased adverse effects.
quetiapine fumarate • Seroquel		
borage	May reduce seizure threshold, increasing risk of seizures.	▪ Discourage use together, especially if pt has seizure history. ▪ Monitor pt for seizure activity.

evening primrose oil **fennel oil** **ginkgo** **St. John's wort** **wormwood**		
capsicum catnip goldenseal **kava** lady's slipper lemon balm melatonin nettle passion flower sassafras skullcap valerian	May cause excessive physical depression, sedation, and impairment. Use of kava may cause coma.	▪ Discourage use together. ▪ Monitor pt for signs and symptoms of increased CNS depression, including sedation, dizziness, ataxia, altered mental status, and respiratory depression.
ginseng ma huang	Because of the CNS stimulant activity of these herbs, discourage use with antipsychotics.	▪ Discourage use together.
nutmeg	May cause a loss of symptom control or interfere with existing therapy for psychiatric illnesses.	▪ Discourage use together. Monitor pt for clinical effect.
sage	May induce seizures.	▪ Discourage use together.

Interacting herbs in **bold type** indicate life-threatening reactions.

◆ Canadian

Herb	Possible effects	Clinical tips
quinapril • Accupril		
agrimony bitter orange celery seed coriander dong quai fennel khella lovage motherwort Queen Anne's lace rosemary (topical) St. John's wort	May increase photosensitivity, adding to risk of sunburn or rash.	▪ Advise pt to wear a sunscreen or protective clothing during sun exposure.
black cohosh	May increase peripheral vasodilation, resulting in hypotension.	▪ Monitor BP closely. ▪ Dosage adjustment may be needed.
capsaicin	May increase risk of cough.	▪ Discourage use together.
goldenseal yohimbe bark	May interfere with drug's action because herb has hypertensive properties.	▪ Monitor pt for clinical effect. ▪ Monitor BP.
licorice	May cause sodium retention and increase BP, interfering with therapeutic effects of ACE inhibitors.	▪ Advise pt of this effect. ▪ Monitor BP.

quinidine • Apo-Quinidine ◆, Cardioquin, Cin-Quin, Novoquinidin ◆, Quinaglute Dura-Tabs, Quinate ◆, Quinidex Extentabs, Quinora

Herb	Interaction	Action
adonis kombé seed lily-of-the-valley	Use together may increase action of herb.	▪ Advise pt against use together unless approved by health care provider. Monitor pt for increased effects such as changes in cardiac rhythm and vital signs and electrolyte abnormalities.
aloe **buckthorn** **cascara sagrada** **Chinese rhubarb** **frangula** **guarana** **licorice** **senna**	May change cardiac rhythm and increase potential for arrhythmias because herb causes hypokalemia.	▪ Monitor pt for signs and symptoms of hypokalemia, including muscle weakness, fatigue, nausea, vomiting, constipation, respiratory depression, and arrhythmias.
belladonna henbane	May increase herbal anticholinergic effects.	▪ Monitor pt for increased adverse effects, including headache, dizziness, confusion, irritability, tachycardia, mydriasis, dry mouth, constipation, urinary retention, and hot, dry skin.
broom	May increase risk of adverse effects.	▪ Monitor pt for increased adverse effects.
digitalis **Indian squill** **squill**	May increase risk of cardiac arrhythmias.	▪ Monitor vital signs and ECG.
jimsonweed	May adversely affect function of CV system.	▪ Advise pt of this effect. ▪ Monitor vital signs and ECG.

Herb	Possible effects	Clinical tips
quinidine *(continued)*		
licorice	May prolong the QT interval. May cause additive effects.	▪ Monitor vital signs and ECG.
ma huang	Increases risk of arrhythmias.	▪ Discourage use together.
oleander scopolia strophanthus	May increase effects of quinidine.	▪ Monitor pt for increased adverse effects, including vertigo, seizures, cardiac arrhythmias, hypotension, respiratory distress, and hematologic abnormalities.
ranitidine • Tritec, Zantac		
blessed thistle bogbean capsicum ginger goldenseal mustard sweet flag true unicorn root yarrow yew	May decrease drug effectiveness because these herbs cause increased acid secretion.	▪ Advise pt of this effect. ▪ Monitor pt for clinical effect.
repaglinide • Prandin		
aloe bilberry leaf bitter melon bladderwrack	May improve glucose control, requiring a reduction of antidiabetics. Some of these herbs may stimulate endogenous insulin release.	▪ Advise pt to consult health care provider before using herbs. ▪ Monitor glucose level. ▪ Monitor pt for signs and symptoms of hypoglycemia, such as dizziness, diaphoresis, confusion, and tachycardia.

burdock dandelion fenugreek garlic ginseng goat's rue gymnema		
angelica broom buchu juniper ma huang	May decrease drug's hypoglycemic effect because of herbs' hyperglycemic properties.	▪ Monitor glucose level. ▪ Monitor pt for signs and symptoms of hyperglycemia (fatigue, polyuria, altered mental status, glucosuria, and ketonuria).
basil bay bee pollen burdock ginkgo biloba ginseng glucomannan horehound marshmallow myrrh sage senega root yarrow	May affect glycemic control and disrupt a previously stable medical regimen.	▪ Monitor glucose level. ▪ Monitor pt for signs and symptoms of hyperglycemia (fatigue, polyuria, polydipsia, wt loss, abdominal pain, altered mental status, tachycardia, hypotension, glucosuria, ketonuria) or hypoglycemia (dizziness, diaphoresis, confusion, tachycardia). ▪ Dosage adjustments may be needed.
bitter melon **fenugreek**	May cause hepatotoxicity.	▪ Hepatic dysfunction may cause increased hypoglycemia caused by decreased drug metabolism.

(continued)

Interacting herbs in **bold type** indicate life-threatening reactions.

◆ Canadian

Herb	Possible effects	Clinical tips
repaglinide *(continued)*		
skullcap **woundwort** **yerba maté**		▪ Monitor LFT values. ▪ Signs and symptoms of liver damage include abdominal pain, fever, malaise, jaundice, dark urine, clay-colored stools, and increased LFT values.
boneset **butterbur** **chaparral** **coltsfoot** **comfrey**	Contains pyrrolizidine alkaloids, which may be hepatotoxic.	▪ Hepatic dysfunction may cause increased hypoglycemia caused by decreased drug metabolism. ▪ Monitor LFT values. ▪ Signs and symptoms of liver damage include abdominal pain, fever, malaise, jaundice, dark urine, clay-colored stools, and increased LFT values.
rifabutin • Mycobutin		
echinacea	May exacerbate HIV infect or AIDS.	▪ Discourage use together.
rifampin (rifampicin) • Rifadin, Rifadin IV, Rimactane, Rofact ◆		
bitter melon **fenugreek** **skullcap** **woundwort** **yerba maté**	May cause hepatotoxicity.	▪ Monitor LFT values. ▪ Signs and symptoms of liver damage include abdominal pain, fever, malaise, jaundice, dark urine, clay-colored stools, and increased LFT values.
boneset **butterbur** **chaparral** **coltsfoot** **comfrey**	Contains pyrrolizidine alkaloids, which may be hepatotoxic.	▪ Signs and symptoms of liver damage include abdominal pain, fever, malaise, jaundice, dark urine, clay-colored stools, and increased LFT values.

echinacea	May increase hepatotoxicity if used with drugs that elevate liver enzyme levels. May exacerbate tuberculosis.	▪ Advise pt of this adverse effect. ▪ Monitor LFT values. ▪ Discourage use together.
fumitory **gossypol** **juniper** **oak bark** **wild ginger** **wintergreen** **yohimbe**	May increase risk of nephrotoxicity or RF.	▪ Inform pt of herb's nephrotoxic potential. ▪ Monitor results of renal function studies.
rifapentine • Priftin		
bitter melon **fenugreek** **skullcap** **woundwort** **yerba maté**	May cause hepatotoxicity.	▪ Monitor LFT values. ▪ Signs and symptoms of liver damage include abdominal pain, fever, malaise, jaundice, dark urine, clay-colored stools, and increased LFT values.
boneset **butterbur** **chaparral** **coltsfoot** **comfrey**	Contains pyrrolizidine alkaloids, which may be hepatotoxic.	▪ Signs and symptoms of liver damage include abdominal pain, fever, malaise, jaundice, dark urine, clay-colored stools, and increased LFT values.
echinacea	May increase hepatotoxicity if used with drugs that elevate liver enzyme levels. May exacerbate tuberculosis.	▪ Advise pt of this adverse effect. ▪ Monitor LFT values. ▪ Discourage use together.

Herb	Possible effects	Clinical tips
risperidone • Risperdal		
agrimony bitter orange celery seed coriander dong quai fennel khella lovage motherwort Queen Anne's lace rosemary (topical) St. John's wort	May increase photosensitivity, adding to risk of sunburn or rash.	▪ Advise pt to wear a sunscreen or protective clothing during sun exposure.
capsicum catnip goldenseal **kava** lady's slipper lemon balm melatonin nettle passion flower sassafras skullcap	May cause excessive physical depression, sedation, and impairment. Use of kava may cause coma.	▪ Discourage use together. ▪ Monitor pt for signs and symptoms of increased CNS depression, including sedation, dizziness, ataxia, altered mental status, and respiratory depression.

valerian		
ginseng ma huang	Herb may act as CNS stimulant.	▪ Discourage use together.
kava	May cause tremors, muscle spasms, or abnormal movements, worsening adverse drug effects.	▪ Advise pt of this effect. ▪ Monitor pt for worsening extrapyramidal movements, tardive dyskinesia, dystonias, and akathisia.
nutmeg	May cause a loss of symptom control or interfere with existing therapy for psychiatric illnesses.	▪ Discourage use together. ▪ Monitor pt for clinical effect.
ritonavir • Norvir		
bitter melon **fenugreek** **skullcap** **woundwort** **yerba maté**	May cause hepatotoxicity.	▪ Monitor LFT values. ▪ Signs and symptoms of liver damage include abdominal pain, fever, malaise, jaundice, dark urine, clay-colored stools, and increased LFT values.
boneset **butterbur** **chaparral** **coltsfoot** **comfrey**	Contains pyrrolizidine alkaloids, which may be hepatotoxic.	▪ Discourage use. ▪ Signs and symptoms of liver damage include abdominal pain, fever, malaise, jaundice, dark urine, clay-colored stools, and increased LFT values.
echinacea	May increase hepatotoxicity if used with drugs that elevate liver enzyme levels. May exacerbate HIV infect or AIDS.	▪ Advise pt of these effects. ▪ Discourage use together.

Herb	Possible effects	Clinical tips
ritonavir *(continued)*		
garlic	May cause severe GI toxicity. May reduce the effectiveness of some drugs used for HIV.	▪ Discourage use together.
St. John's wort	Reduces indinavir levels by more than 50%. May have similar effects with other protease inhibitors.	▪ Discourage use together.
rizatriptan benzoate • Maxalt, Maxalt-MLT		
bugleweed goldenseal ma huang Scotch broom witch hazel	May increase vasoconstriction.	▪ Monitor pt for increased vasospastic reactions.
feverfew	May increase BP and heart rate to dangerous levels.	▪ Advise pt of this effect. ▪ Monitor vital signs closely.
horehound St. John's wort	May enhance serotonergic effects.	▪ Discourage use together. ▪ Monitor pt for weakness, hyperreflexia, and incoordination.
rofecoxib • Vioxx		
agrimony bitter orange celery seed coriander dong quai	May increase photosensitivity, adding to risk of sunburn or rash.	▪ Advise pt to wear a sunscreen or protective clothing during sun exposure.

fennel khella lovage motherwort Queen Anne's lace rosemary (topical) St. John's wort		
angelica root anise bilberry borage seed oil danshen devil's claw dong quai echinacea feverfew garlic ginger ginkgo biloba horse chestnut licorice passion flower red clover	May increase risk of bleeding because of coumarin or coumarin derivatives in the herb or because of the herb's antiplatelet activity.	▪ Monitor pt for signs and symptoms of increased bleeding, including bruising, petechiae, bleeding gums, epistaxis, prolonged bleeding after injury, melena, GI bleeding, hematuria, and hematemesis. ▪ Monitor results of hematologic studies and coagulation studies. ▪ Advise pt to consult health care provider before using herb.
bitter melon **fenugreek**	May cause hepatotoxicity.	▪ Monitor LFT values. ▪ Signs and symptoms of liver damage

(continued)

Herb	Possible effects	Clinical tips
rofecoxib *(continued)*		
skullcap **woundwort** **yerba maté**		include abdominal pain, fever, malaise, jaundice, dark urine, clay-colored stools, and increased LFT values.
boneset **butterbur** **chaparral** **coltsfoot** **comfrey**	Contains pyrrolizidine alkaloids, which may be hepatotoxic.	▪ Discourage use together. ▪ Signs and symptoms of liver damage include abdominal pain, fever, malaise, jaundice, dark urine, clay-colored stools, and increased LFT values.
capsicum	Stimulates GI secretions to help protect against NSAID-induced GI irritation.	▪ May be used for therapeutic advantage.
coffea arabica cola gossypol uva-ursi	May cause increased adverse GI effects.	▪ Inform pt of increased risk of adverse GI effects.
meadowsweet white willow	May increase risk of bleeding because of salicylates in the herb.	▪ Monitor pt for signs and symptoms of increased bleeding, including bruising, petechiae, bleeding gums, epistaxis, prolonged bleeding after injury, melena, GI bleeding, hematuria, and hematemesis. ▪ Monitor results of hematologic studies and coagulation studies.
wild yam	May decrease drug's anti-inflammatory effect.	▪ Monitor pt for clinical effects.

rosiglitazone • Avandia

Herbs	Interaction	Nursing considerations
aloe bilberry leaf bitter melon bladderwrack burdock dandelion fenugreek garlic ginseng goat's rue gymnema	May improve glucose control, requiring a reduction of antidiabetic dose. May stimulate endogenous insulin release.	▪ Advise pt to consult health care provider before using herbs. ▪ Monitor glucose level. ▪ Monitor pt for signs and symptoms of hypoglycemia (dizziness, diaphoresis, confusion, and tachycardia).
angelica broom buchu juniper ma huang	May decrease drug's hypoglycemic effect because of herb's hyperglycemic properties.	▪ Monitor glucose level. ▪ Monitor pt for signs and symptoms of hyperglycemia (fatigue, polyuria, polydipsia, wt loss, abdominal pain, altered mental status, tachycardia, hypotension, glucosuria, and ketonuria).
basil bay bee pollen burdock ginkgo biloba ginseng glucomannan horehound marshmallow	May affect glycemic control and disrupt a previously stable medical regimen.	▪ Monitor glucose level and adjust drug dosage if needed. ▪ Monitor pt for signs of hyperglycemia (polyuria, polydipsia, wt loss, tachycardia, hypotension, glucosuria, ketonuria) or hypoglycemia (diaphoresis, tachycardia).

Herb	Possible effects	Clinical tips
rosiglitazone *(continued)*		
myrrh sage senega root yarrow	May affect glycemic control and disrupt a previously stable medical regimen.	▪ Monitor glucose level and adjust drug dosage if needed. ▪ Monitor pt for signs of hyperglycemia (polyuria, polydipsia, wt loss, tachycardia, hypotension, glucosuria, ketonuria) or hypoglycemia (diaphoresis, tachycardia).
bitter melon **fenugreek** **skullcap** **woundwort** **yerba maté**	May cause hepatotoxicity.	▪ Monitor LFT values. ▪ Signs and symptoms of liver damage include abdominal pain, fever, malaise, jaundice, dark urine, clay-colored stools, and increased LFT values.
boneset **butterbur** **chaparral** **coltsfoot** **comfrey**	May cause hepatotoxicity.	▪ Monitor LFT values. ▪ Signs and symptoms of liver damage include abdominal pain, fever, malaise, jaundice, dark urine, clay-colored stools, and increased LFT values.
saquinavir • Fortovase, Invirase		
bitter melon **fenugreek** **skullcap** **woundwort** **yerba maté**	May cause hepatotoxicity.	▪ Monitor LFT values. ▪ Signs and symptoms of liver damage include abdominal pain, fever, malaise, jaundice, dark urine, clay-colored stools, and increased LFT values.
boneset **butterbur**	Contains pyrrolizidine alkaloids, which may be hepatotoxic.	▪ Discourage use together. ▪ Signs and symptoms of liver damage include abdominal pain,

Herb	Effect	Nursing considerations
chaparral **coltsfoot** **comfrey**		fever, malaise, jaundice, dark urine, clay-colored stools, and increased LFT values.
echinacea	May increase hepatotoxicity if used with drugs that elevate liver enzyme levels. May exacerbate HIV infect or AIDS.	▪ Advise pt of these effects. ▪ Discourage use together.
garlic	May cause severe GI toxicity. May reduce the effectiveness of some drugs used for HIV.	▪ Discourage use together.
St. John's wort	Reduces indinavir levels by more than 50%. May have similar effects with other protease inhibitors.	▪ Discourage use together.
selegiline hydrochloride • Eldepryl		
brewer's yeast cola ephedra green tea Scotch broom St. John's wort	May cause hypertensive crisis.	▪ Discourage use together. ▪ Monitor BP. ▪ Monitor pt for headache, dizziness, palpitations, nausea, and chest tightness.
cacao tree	May have vasopressor effects.	▪ Discourage use together. ▪ Monitor vital signs and ECG.
ginkgo nutmeg parsley	May potentiate drug's action.	▪ Discourage use together. ▪ Monitor pt for increased adverse effects.

Herb	Possible effects	Clinical tips
selegiline hydrochloride *(continued)*		
passion flower sweet flower	May potentiate drug's action.	▪ Discourage use together. ▪ Monitor pt for increased adverse effects.
ginseng	May precipitate adverse reactions, including headache, tremors, and mania.	▪ Discourage use together.
kava	May cause tremors, muscle spasms, or abnormal movements. May decrease drug's effect.	▪ Monitor pt for clinical effect. ▪ Discourage use together.
sertraline • Zoloft		
5-HTP **SAMe**	May cause serotonin syn.	▪ Discourage use together. ▪ Monitor pt for signs and symptoms of serotonin syn, including nausea, hypotension, HTN, excitation, mental status changes, hyperpyrexia, and coma.
ginkgo	May reduce sexual adverse effects of SSRIs in both men and women.	▪ Advise pt of this effect.
St. John's wort	May cause serotonin syn. May cause sedative-hypnotic intoxication.	▪ Discourage use together. ▪ Advise pt switching from SSRI to St. John's wort to wait a few weeks for the SSRI to wash out of his system before it's safe to start taking the herb. The exact time needed depends on which SSRI was used. ▪ Advise pt to consult health care provider before using herb.
yohimbe	May cause serotonin syn.	▪ Discourage use together.

sildenafil • Viagra		
aloe **buckthorn** **cascara sagrada** **Chinese rhubarb** **frangula** **guarana** **licorice** **senna**	May change cardiac rhythm and increase potential for arrhythmias because herb causes hypokalemia.	▪ Monitor pt for signs and symptoms of hypokalemia, including muscle weakness, fatigue, nausea, vomiting, constipation, respiratory depression, and arrhythmias.
black cohosh *Coleus forskohlii*	Relaxes blood vessels and may have unpredictable effects on BP if combined with beta blockers.	▪ Discourage use together.
ma huang **squill**	Increases risk of arrhythmias.	▪ Discourage use together.
simvastatin (synvinolin) • Zocor		
bitter melon **fenugreek** **skullcap** **woundwort** **yerba maté**	May cause hepatotoxicity.	▪ Monitor LFT values. ▪ Signs and symptoms of liver damage include abdominal pain, fever, malaise, jaundice, dark urine, clay-colored stools, and increased LFT values.
boneset **butterbur** **chaparral**	Contains pyrrolizidine alkaloids, which may be hepatotoxic.	▪ Discourage use together. ▪ Signs and symptoms of liver damage include abdominal pain, fever, malaise, jaundice, dark urine, *(continued)*

Herb	Possible effects	Clinical tips
simvastatin (synvinolin) *(continued)*		
coltsfoot **comfrey**		clay-colored stools, and increased LFT values.
echinacea	May increase hepatotoxicity if used with drugs that elevate liver enzyme levels.	▪ Monitor LFT values.
garlic	May have additive lipid-lowering properties.	▪ May be used for therapeutic advantage.
pectin	May decrease the effectiveness of HMG-CoA reductase inhibitors.	▪ Discourage use together. ▪ Monitor pt for clinical response.
red yeast rice	Contains similar components to those of statin drugs, increasing risk of adverse events or toxicity.	▪ Advise pt to avoid using together if possible. ▪ Monitor pt for signs and symptoms of increased adverse effects such as myopathy and rhabdomyolysis (increased creatinine kinase level, muscle aches, weakness) or increased LFT values.
St. John's wort	May decrease blood levels of various drugs in the statin family.	▪ Monitor pt for clinical response.
sotalol • Betapace		
aloe **buckthorn** **cascara sagrada** **Chinese rhubarb** **frangula**	May change cardiac rhythm and increase potential for arrhythmias because herb causes hypokalemia.	▪ Monitor pt for signs and symptoms of hypokalemia, including muscle weakness, fatigue, nausea, vomiting, constipation, respiratory depression, and arrhythmias.

Herb	Effect	Nursing considerations
guarana **licorice** **senna**		
black cohosh *Coleus forskohlii*	Relaxes blood vessels and may have unpredictable effects on BP if combined with beta blockers.	▪ Advise pt of this effect. ▪ Monitor BP closely.
lily-of-the-valley	May increase risk of bradycardia or heart block.	▪ Monitor vital signs and ECG closely.
ma huang	Increases risk of arrhythmias.	▪ Discourage use together.
stavudine • Zerit		
bitter melon **fenugreek** **skullcap** **woundwort** **yerba maté**	May cause hepatotoxicity.	▪ Monitor LFT values. ▪ Signs and symptoms of liver damage include abdominal pain, fever, malaise, jaundice, dark urine, clay-colored stools, and increased LFT values.
boneset **butterbur** **chaparral** **coltsfoot** **comfrey**	Contains pyrrolizidine alkaloids, which may be hepatotoxic.	▪ Discourage use together. ▪ Signs and symptoms of liver damage include abdominal pain, fever, malaise, jaundice, dark urine, clay-colored stools, and increased LFT values.
echinacea	May increase hepatotoxicity if used with drugs that elevate liver enzyme levels. May exacerbate HIV infect or AIDS.	▪ Advise pt of these effects. ▪ Discourage use together.

Herb	Possible effects	Clinical tips
stavudine *(continued)*		
fumitory **gossypol** **juniper** **oak bark** **wild ginger** **wintergreen** **yohimbe**	May increase risk of nephrotoxicity or RF. Impaired renal function may limit drug excretion.	▪ Inform pt of herb's nephrotoxic potential. ▪ Monitor results of renal function studies. ▪ Monitor pt for signs and symptoms of toxicity, such as peripheral neuropathy and neurotoxicity, GI complaints, pancreatitis, and hematologic abnormalities.
snakeroot	May increase risk of renal problems because one component of snakeroot, aristolochic acid, has nephrotoxic properties.	▪ Discourage use together because of herb's toxic and carcinogenic potential.
sucralfate • Carafate		
blessed thistle bogbean capsicum ginger goldenseal mustard sweet flag true unicorn root yarrow yew	May decrease effectiveness because herb causes increased acid secretion.	▪ Advise pt of this effect. ▪ Monitor pt for clinical effect. ▪ Discourage use together unless approved by health care provider.
fumitory **gossypol**	May increase risk of nephrotoxicity or RF. Pt with renal insufficiency is at increased	▪ Inform pt of herb's nephrotoxic potential. ▪ Monitor results of renal function studies.

juniper **oak bark** **wild ginger** **wintergreen** **yohimbe**	risk for aluminum toxicity.	
snakeroot	May increase risk of renal problems because one component of snakeroot, aristolochic acid, has nephrotoxic properties.	▪ Discourage use together because of herb's toxic and carcinogenic potential.
tamoxifen • Novaldex, Novaldex-D ◆, Novo-Tamoxifen ◆, Tamofen ◆, Tamone ◆		
bitter melon **fenugreek** **skullcap** **woundwort** **yerba maté**	May cause hepatotoxicity.	▪ Monitor LFT values. ▪ Signs and symptoms of liver damage include abdominal pain, fever, malaise, jaundice, dark urine, clay-colored stools, and increased LFT values.
boneset **butterbur** **chaparral** **coltsfoot** **comfrey**	Contains pyrrolizidine alkaloids, which may be hepatotoxic.	▪ Signs and symptoms of liver damage include abdominal pain, fever, malaise, jaundice, dark urine, clay-colored stools, and increased LFT values.
echinacea	May increase hepatotoxicity if used with drugs that elevate liver enzyme levels.	▪ Advise pt of this effect. ▪ Monitor LFT values.
ginger	May decrease nausea caused by chemo.	▪ May be used for clinical effect.
soy	May decrease drug effects.	▪ Advise pt of potential interaction. ▪ Monitor pt for clinical effect.

Herb	Possible effects	Clinical tips
tamoxifen *(continued)*		
yew	May potentiate myelosuppression and interactions with other chemo drugs.	▪ Monitor results of hematologic studies. ▪ Monitor pt for increased adverse effects. ▪ Discourage use together unless approved by health care provider.
temazepam • Restoril		
capsicum catnip goldenseal **kava** lady's slipper lemon balm melatonin nettle passion flower sassafras skullcap valerian	May cause excessive physical depression, sedation, and impairment. Use of kava may cause coma.	▪ Discourage use together. ▪ Monitor pt for signs and symptoms of increased CNS depression, including sedation, dizziness, ataxia, altered mental status, and respiratory depression.
echinacea	May increase hepatotoxicity if used with drugs that elevate liver enzyme levels.	▪ Advise pt of this effect. ▪ Monitor LFT values.
linden	May increase adverse effects of benzodiazepine because herb contains similar components.	▪ Discourage use of excessive amounts of herb.

Herb	Interaction	Nursing considerations
tetracycline • Achromycin V, Apo-Tetra ◆, Novo-Tetra ◆, Nu-Tetra ◆, Panmycin, Sumycin		
agrimony bitter orange celery seed coriander dong quai fennel khella lovage motherwort Queen Anne's lace rosemary (topical) St. John's wort	May increase photosensitivity, adding to risk of sunburn or rash.	▪ Advise pt to wear a sunscreen or protective clothing during sun exposure.
echinacea	May increase hepatotoxicity if used with drugs that elevate liver enzyme levels. May exacerbate tuberculosis.	▪ Discourage use of herb.
theophylline • Accurbron, Aerolate SR, Aquaphyllin, Asmalix, Bronkodyl, Elixophyllin, Lanophyllin, Quibron-T Dividose, Respid, Slo-Phyllin, Theo-24, Theoclear-80, Theo-Dur, Theolair, Theospan-SR, Theostat 80, Theovent Long-Acting, Uni-Dur, Uniphyl		
cacao tree	May inhibit theophylline metabolism.	▪ Discourage ingestion of large amounts of cocoa while taking theophylline.
capsicum	May increase the absorption of theophylline, possibly leading to higher serum levels or toxicity.	▪ Discourage use together. ▪ Theophylline has a low therapeutic index.

Herb	Possible effects	Clinical tips
theophylline *(continued)*		
cayenne ipriflavone	May increase risk of theophylline toxicity.	▪ Monitor theophylline levels. ▪ Monitor pt for signs and symptoms of theophylline toxicity, including tachycardia, nausea, vomiting, diarrhea, restlessness, headache, agitation, palpitations, and arrhythmias.
digitalis **Indian squill** **squill**	May increase risk of cardiac arrhythmias.	▪ Monitor vital signs and ECG. ▪ Discourage use together unless approved by health care provider.
ephedra green tea guarana	May cause additive CNS and CV effects.	▪ Monitor pt for changes in BP and heart rate, insomnia, nervousness, tremors, and headache. ▪ Discourage use of herb and other sources of caffeine.
St. John's wort	Induces cytochrome P450 enzyme system and may lower theophylline levels.	▪ Monitor theophylline levels. ▪ Monitor pt for decreased clinical effects.
ticlopidine • Ticlid		
angelica root anise bilberry borage seed oil danshen devil's claw dong quai echinacea feverfew garlic	May increase risk of bleeding because of coumarin or coumarin derivatives in the herbs.	▪ Monitor pt for signs and symptoms of increased bleeding, including bruising, petechiae, bleeding gums, epistaxis, prolonged bleeding after injury, melena, GI bleeding, hematuria, and hematemesis. ▪ Monitor results of hematologic studies and coagulation studies. ▪ Advise pt to consult health care provider before using herb.

ginger ginkgo biloba horse chestnut licorice passion flower red clover		
astragalus vitamin E–containing herbs (e.g., sunflower seeds)	May potentiate anticoagulant effects.	▪ Monitor PT and INR. ▪ Dosage adjustment may be needed.
bilberry	Decreases platelet aggregation.	▪ Monitor results of hematologic studies and coagulation studies.
borage seed oil	May increase coagulation time because of y-linoleic acid in herb.	▪ Monitor pt for signs and symptoms of increased bleeding, including bruising, petechiae, bleeding gums, epistaxis, prolonged bleeding after injury, melena, GI bleeding, hematuria, and hematemesis. ▪ Monitor results of hematologic studies and coagulation studies.
bromelain clove ginkgo biloba onion turmeric	May increase risk of bleeding because of antiplatelet activity of herb.	▪ Monitor pt for signs and symptoms of increased bleeding, including bruising, petechiae, bleeding gums, epistaxis, prolonged bleeding after injury, melena, GI bleeding, hematuria, and hematemesis. ▪ Monitor results of hematologic studies and coagulation studies.

Herb	Possible effects	Clinical tips
ticlopidine *(continued)*		
capsicum feverfew	Decreases platelet aggregation and increases fibrolytic activity, prolonging bleeding time.	▪ Monitor pt for signs and symptoms of increased bleeding, including bruising, petechiae, bleeding gums, epistaxis, prolonged bleeding after injury, melena, GI bleeding, hematuria, and hematemesis. ▪ Monitor results of hematologic studies and coagulation studies.
echinacea	May increase bleeding time without increasing INR.	▪ Monitor pt for signs and symptoms of increased bleeding, including bruising, petechiae, bleeding gums, epistaxis, prolonged bleeding after injury, melena, GI bleeding, hematuria, and hematemesis.
ginger	Inhibits platelet aggregation by antagonizing thromboxane synthetase and enhancing prostacyclin, leading to prolonged bleeding time.	▪ Monitor pt for signs and symptoms of increased bleeding, including bruising, petechiae, bleeding gums, epistaxis, prolonged bleeding after injury, melena, GI bleeding, hematuria, and hematemesis. ▪ Monitor results of hematologic studies and coagulation studies.
grapeseed	Increases drug effects and INR because of tocopherol content of herb.	▪ Monitor pt for signs and symptoms of increased bleeding, including bruising, petechiae, bleeding gums, epistaxis, prolonged bleeding after injury, melena, GI bleeding, hematuria, and hematemesis. ▪ Monitor results of hematologic studies and coagulation studies.

Herb	Effect	Nursing considerations
meadowsweet white willow	May increase risk of bleeding because of salicylates in herb.	▪ Monitor pt for signs and symptoms of increased bleeding, including bruising, petechiae, bleeding gums, epistaxis, prolonged bleeding after injury, melena, GI bleeding, hematuria, and hematemesis. ▪ Monitor results of hematologic studies and coagulation studies.
timolol maleate • Apo-Timol ◆, Blocadren		
black cohosh *Coleus forskohlii*	Relaxes blood vessels and may have unpredictable effects on BP if combined with beta blockers.	▪ Advise pt of this effect. ▪ Monitor BP closely.
ephedra	May increase BP because of unopposed sympathetic stimulation.	▪ Monitor pt for changes in BP and heart rate, arrhythmias, and shortness of breath.
goldenseal yohimbe bark	May interfere with the drug's action because these herbs have hypertensive properties.	▪ Advise pt of this effect. ▪ Monitor BP.
licorice	May increase sodium, chloride, and H_2O retention, resulting in BP increase.	▪ Monitor BP.
lily-of-the-valley	May increase risk of bradycardia or heart block.	▪ Monitor vital signs and ECG closely.
tramadol • Ultram		
bitter melon **fenugreek** **skullcap** **woundwort** **yerba maté**	May cause hepatotoxicity. Hepatic dysfunction may prolong drug effects.	▪ Discourage use together. ▪ Monitor LFT values. ▪ Signs and symptoms of liver damage include abdominal pain, fever, malaise, jaundice, dark urine, clay-colored stools, and increased LFT values.

Herb	Possible effects	Clinical tips
tramadol *(continued)*		
boneset **butterbur** **chaparral** **coltsfoot** **comfrey**	Contains pyrrolizidine alkaloids, which may be hepatotoxic. Hepatic dysfunction may prolong drug effects.	▪ Discourage use together. ▪ Signs and symptoms of liver damage include abdominal pain, fever, malaise, jaundice, dark urine, clay-colored stools, and increased LFT values.
borage **evening primrose oil** **fennel oil** **ginkgo** **St. John's wort** **wormwood**	May reduce seizure threshold, increasing risk of seizures.	▪ Discourage use together, especially if pt has seizure history. ▪ Monitor pt for seizure activity.
capsicum catnip goldenseal **kava** lady's slipper lemon balm melatonin nettle passion flower sassafras skullcap valerian	May cause excessive physical depression, sedation, and impairment. Use of kava may cause coma.	▪ Discourage use together. ▪ Monitor pt for signs and symptoms of increased CNS depression, including sedation, dizziness, ataxia, altered mental status, and respiratory depression.

fumitory **gossypol** **juniper** **oak bark** **wild ginger** **wintergreen** **yohimbe**	May increase risk of nephrotoxicity or RF. Renal dysfunction may prolong drug effects.	▪ Advise pt of herb's nephrotoxic potential. ▪ Monitor results of renal function studies. ▪ Discourage use together.
sage	May induce seizures.	▪ Discourage use together.
snakeroot	May increase risk of renal problems because one component of snakeroot, aristolochic acid, has nephrotoxic properties.	▪ Discourage use together because of herb's toxic and carcinogenic potential.
triazolam • Apo-Triazo ◆, Halcion, Novo-Triolam ◆		
capsicum catnip goldenseal **kava** lady's slipper lemon balm melatonin nettle passion flower sassafras skullcap valerian	May cause excessive physical depression, sedation, and impairment. Use of kava may cause coma.	▪ Discourage use together. ▪ Monitor pt for signs and symptoms of increased CNS depression, including sedation, dizziness, ataxia, altered mental status, and respiratory depression.
echinacea	May increase hepatotoxicity if used with drugs that elevate liver enzyme levels.	▪ Advise pt of this effect. ▪ Monitor LFT values.

Herb	Possible effects	Clinical tips
triazolam *(continued)*		
linden	May increase side effects of benzodiazepine because herb contains similar components.	▪ Advise pt to avoid excessive amounts of herb.
urokinase • Abbokinase, Abbokinase Open-Cath		
angelica root anise bilberry borage seed oil danshen devil's claw dong quai echinacea feverfew garlic ginger ginkgo biloba horse chestnut licorice passion flower red clover	May increase risk of bleeding because of coumarin or coumarin derivatives in the herb.	▪ Monitor pt for signs and symptoms of increased bleeding, including bruising, petechiae, bleeding gums, epistaxis, prolonged bleeding after injury, melena, GI bleeding, hematuria, and hematemesis. ▪ Monitor results of hematologic studies and coagulation studies.
astragalus vitamin E–containing	May potentiate anticoagulant effects.	▪ Monitor PT and INR.

herbs (e.g., sunflower seeds)		
bilberry	May decrease platelet aggregation.	▪ Monitor results of hematologic studies and coagulation studies.
borage seed oil	May increase coagulation time because of y-linoleic acid in the herb.	▪ Monitor pt for signs and symptoms of increased bleeding, including bruising, petechiae, bleeding gums, epistaxis, prolonged bleeding after injury, melena, GI bleeding, hematuria, and hematemesis. ▪ Monitor results of hematologic studies and coagulation studies.
bromelain clove ginkgo biloba onion turmeric	May increase risk of bleeding because of antiplatelet activity of the herb.	▪ Monitor pt for signs and symptoms of increased bleeding, including bruising, petechiae, bleeding gums, epistaxis, prolonged bleeding after injury, melena, GI bleeding, hematuria, and hematemesis. ▪ Monitor results of hematologic studies and coagulation studies.
capsicum feverfew	May decrease platelet aggregation and increase fibrolytic activity, prolonging bleeding time.	▪ Monitor pt for signs and symptoms of increased bleeding, including bruising, petechiae, bleeding gums, epistaxis, prolonged bleeding after injury, melena, GI bleeding, hematuria, and hematemesis. ▪ Monitor results of hematologic studies and coagulation studies.
echinacea	May increase bleeding time without increasing INR.	▪ Monitor pt for signs and symptoms of increased bleeding, including bruising, petechiae, bleeding *(continued)*

Herb	Possible effects	Clinical tips
urokinase *(continued)*		
echinacea *(continued)*		gums, epistaxis, prolonged bleeding after injury, melena, GI bleeding, hematuria, and hematemesis.
ginger	May inhibit platelet aggregation by antagonizing thromboxane synthetase and enhancing prostacyclin, leading to prolonged bleeding time.	▪ Monitor pt for signs and symptoms of increased bleeding, including bruising, petechiae, bleeding gums, epistaxis, prolonged bleeding after injury, melena, GI bleeding, hematuria, and hematemesis. ▪ Monitor results of hematologic studies and coagulation studies.
grapeseed	May increase drug effects and INR because of tocopherol content of herb.	▪ Monitor pt for signs and symptoms of increased bleeding, including bruising, petechiae, bleeding gums, epistaxis, prolonged bleeding after injury, melena, GI bleeding, hematuria, and hematemesis. ▪ Monitor results of hematologic studies and coagulation studies.
meadowsweet white willow	May increase risk of bleeding because of salicylates in the herb.	▪ Monitor pt for signs and symptoms of increased bleeding, including bruising, petechiae, bleeding gums, epistaxis, prolonged bleeding after injury, melena, GI bleeding, hematuria, and hematemesis. ▪ Monitor results of hematologic studies and coagulation studies.
valacyclovir • Valtrex		
fumitory **gossypol**	May increase risk of nephrotoxicity or RF. Increases risk of drug-induced renal dys-	▪ Pt may be unaware of the nephrotoxic potential of these herbs. ▪ Monitor results of renal function studies.

Herb	Interaction	Nursing considerations
juniper **oak bark** **wild ginger** **wintergreen** **yohimbe**	function and adverse CNS effects.	
snakeroot	May increase risk of renal problems because one component of snakeroot, aristolochic acid, has nephrotoxic properties.	▪ Discourage use together because of herb's toxic and carcinogenic potential.
valganciclovir • Valcyte		
echinacea	May worsen HIV infect or AIDS.	▪ Advise pt with HIV or AIDS to avoid this herb.
fumitory **gossypol** **juniper** **oak bark** **wild ginger** **wintergreen** **yohimbe**	May increase risk of nephrotoxicity or RF. May increase drug's adverse effects because drug is excreted via renal elimination.	▪ Pt may be unaware of herb's nephrotoxic potential. ▪ Monitor results of renal function studies. ▪ Monitor pt for increased adverse effects such as peripheral neuropathy and hematologic abnormalities.
snakeroot	May increase risk of renal problems because one component of snakeroot, aristolochic acid, has nephrotoxic properties.	▪ Discourage use together because of herb's toxic and carcinogenic potential.
valsartan • Diovan		
black cohosh	May increase peripheral vasodilation, resulting in hypotension.	▪ Monitor BP closely. ▪ Dosage adjustment may be needed.

Herb	Possible effects	Clinical tips
valsartan *(continued)*		
goldenseal yohimbe bark	May interfere with the drug's action because these herbs have hypertensive properties.	▪ Monitor pt for clinical effect. ▪ Monitor BP.
licorice	May increase sodium, chloride, and H_2O retention, resulting in BP increase.	▪ Monitor BP.
vancomycin hydrochloride • Vancocin, Vancoled		
fumitory **gossypol** **juniper** **oak bark** **wild ginger** **wintergreen** **yohimbe**	May increase risk of nephrotoxicity or RF.	▪ Advise pt of herb's nephrotoxic potential. ▪ Monitor results of renal function studies.
snakeroot	May increase risk of renal problems because one component of snakeroot, aristolochic acid, has nephrotoxic properties.	▪ Discourage use together because of herb's toxic and carcinogenic potential.
venlafaxine • Effexor, Effexor XR		
borage **evening primrose oil** **fennel oil** **ginkgo** **St. John's wort** **wormwood**	May reduce seizure threshold, increasing risk of seizures.	▪ Discourage use together, especially if pt has seizure history. ▪ Monitor pt for seizure activity.

capsicum ephedra Scotch broom yohimbe	May cause additive stimulation.	▪ Discourage use together. ▪ Monitor pt for increased adverse effects.
sage	May induce seizures.	▪ Discourage use together.
St. John's wort	Herb has an inhib effect on both MAO inhibitors and reuptake of serotonin.	▪ Discourage use together. ▪ Monitor pt for signs and symptoms of serotonin syn, including nausea, hypotension, HTN, excitation, mental status changes, myoclonus, seizures, hyperpyrexia, and coma.

verapamil hydrochloride • Apo-Verap ◆, Calan, Isoptin, Novo-Veramil ◆, Nu-Verap ◆

aloe **buckthorn** **cascara sagrada** **Chinese rhubarb** **frangula** **guarana** **licorice** **senna**	May cause a change in cardiac rhythm and increase the potential for arrhythmias because of hypokalemia caused by use of these herbs.	▪ Monitor potassium levels. ▪ Monitor pt for signs and symptoms of hypokalemia, including muscle weakness, fatigue, nausea, vomiting, constipation, respiratory depression, and arrhythmias.
black cohosh	Increases peripheral vasodilation, resulting in hypotension.	▪ Monitor BP closely. ▪ Dosage adjustment may be needed.
cat's claw chicory	May increase antianginal effect.	▪ Advise pt to consult health care provider before taking herb.

Herb	Possible effects	Clinical tips
verapamil hydrochloride *(continued)*		
ginger	May increase calcium uptake by the myocardium, leading to altered drug effects.	▪ Monitor pt for therapeutic effect. ▪ Discourage use together.
goldenseal yohimbe bark	May interfere with the drug's action because these herbs have hypertensive properties.	▪ Monitor pt for clinical effect. ▪ Monitor BP.
licorice	May increase sodium, chloride, and H_2O retention, resulting in BP increase.	▪ Monitor BP.
lily-of-the-valley	May increase risk of bradycardia or heart block.	▪ Monitor vital signs and ECG closely.
ma huang	Increases risk of arrhythmias.	▪ Discourage use together.
yerba maté	May decrease clearance of yerba maté methylxanthines and cause toxicity.	▪ Advise pt of this effect. ▪ Monitor pt for increased CNS stimulation.
warfarin sodium • Coumadin, Warfilone ◆		
angelica root anise bilberry borage seed oil danshen devil's claw dong quai echinacea feverfew	May increase risk of bleeding because of coumarin or coumarin derivatives in the herb.	▪ Monitor pt for signs and symptoms of increased bleeding, including bruising, petechiae, bleeding gums, epistaxis, prolonged bleeding after injury, melena, GI bleeding, hematuria, and hematemesis. ▪ Monitor results of hematologic studies and coagulation studies.

garlic ginger ginkgo biloba horse chestnut licorice passion flower red clover		
astragalus vitamin E–containing herbs (e.g., sunflower seeds)	May potentiate anticoagulant effects.	▪ Monitor PT and INR.
bilberry	May decrease platelet aggregation.	▪ Monitor results of hematologic studies and coagulation studies.
borage seed oil	May increase coagulation time because of γ-linoleic acid in the herb.	▪ Monitor pt for signs and symptoms of increased bleeding, including bruising, petechiae, bleeding gums, epistaxis, prolonged bleeding after injury, melena, GI bleeding, hematuria, and hematemesis. ▪ Monitor results of hematologic studies and coagulation studies.
bromelain clove ginkgo biloba motherwort	May increase risk of bleeding because of antiplatelet activity of the herb.	▪ Monitor pt for signs and symptoms of increased bleeding, including bruising, petechiae, bleeding gums, epistaxis, prolonged bleeding after injury, melena, GI bleeding, hematuria, and hematemesis.

(continued)

Herb	Possible effects	Clinical tips
warfarin sodium *(continued)*		
onion turmeric		▪ Monitor results of hematologic studies and coagulation studies.
capsicum feverfew	May decrease platelet aggregation and increase fibrolytic activity, prolonging bleeding time.	▪ Monitor pt for signs and symptoms of increased bleeding, including bruising, petechiae, bleeding gums, epistaxis, prolonged bleeding after injury, melena, GI bleeding, hematuria, and hematemesis. ▪ Monitor results of hematologic studies and coagulation studies.
echinacea	May increase bleeding time without increasing INR.	▪ Monitor pt for signs and symptoms of increased bleeding, including bruising, petechiae, bleeding gums, epistaxis, prolonged bleeding after injury, melena, GI bleeding, hematuria, and hematemesis.
ginger	May inhibit platelet aggregation by antagonizing thromboxane synthetase and enhancing prostacyclin, leading to prolonged bleeding time.	▪ Monitor pt for signs and symptoms of increased bleeding, including bruising, petechiae, bleeding gums, epistaxis, prolonged bleeding after injury, melena, GI bleeding, hematuria, and hematemesis. ▪ Monitor results of hematologic studies and coagulation studies.
grapeseed	May increase drug effects and INR because of tocopherol content of herb.	▪ Monitor pt for signs and symptoms of increased bleeding, including bruising, petechiae, bleeding gums, epistaxis, prolonged bleeding after injury, melena, GI bleeding, hematuria, and hematemesis.

		▪ Monitor results of hematologic studies and coagulation studies.
meadowsweet white willow	May increase risk of bleeding because of salicylates in the herb.	▪ Monitor pt for signs and symptoms of increased bleeding, including bruising, petechiae, bleeding gums, epistaxis, prolonged bleeding after injury, melena, GI bleeding, hematuria, and hematemesis. ▪ Monitor results of hematologic studies and coagulation studies.
zidovudine (azidothymidine, AZT) • Apo-Zidovudine ◆, Novo-AZT ◆, Retrovir		
bitter melon **fenugreek** **skullcap** **woundwort** **yerba maté**	May cause hepatotoxicity.	▪ Monitor LFT values. Signs and symptoms of liver damage include abdominal pain, fever, malaise, jaundice, dark urine, clay-colored stools, and increased LFT values.
boneset **butterbur** **chaparral** **coltsfoot** **comfrey**	Contains pyrrolizidine alkaloids, which may be hepatotoxic.	▪ Discourage use. Signs and symptoms of liver damage include abdominal pain, fever, malaise, jaundice, dark urine, clay-colored stools, and increased LFT values.
echinacea	May increase hepatotoxicity if used with drugs that elevate liver enzyme levels. May exacerbate HIV infect or AIDS.	▪ Advise pt of these effects. Discourage use together.
fumitory **gossypol** **juniper**	May increase risk of nephrotoxicity or RF. Impaired renal function may limit drug excretion.	▪ Pt may be unaware of the nephrotoxic potential of these herbs. ▪ Monitor results of renal function studies.

Herb	Possible effects	Clinical tips
zidovudine (azidothymidine, AZT) *(continued)*		
oak bark **wild ginger** **wintergreen** **yohimbe**	May increase risk of nephrotoxicity or RF. Impaired renal function may limit drug excretion.	▪ Pt may be unaware of the nephrotoxic potential of these herbs. ▪ Monitor results of renal function studies.
snakeroot	May increase risk of renal problems because one component of snakeroot, aristolochic acid, has nephrotoxic properties.	▪ Discourage use together because of herb's toxic and carcinogenic potential.
zolmitriptan • Zomig		
bugleweed goldenseal ma huang Scotch broom witch hazel	May increase vasoconstriction.	▪ Monitor pt for increased vasospastic reactions.
feverfew	May increase BP and heart rate to dangerous levels if combined with drug.	▪ Advise pt of this effect. ▪ Monitor vital signs closely.
St. John's wort	May have MAO inhib properties, causing increased adverse drug effects.	▪ Monitor pt for increased adverse effects such as HTN, pain or heaviness in chest, arrhythmias, and warm or cold sensations.
zolpidem • Ambien		
capsicum catnip goldenseal **kava**	May cause excessive physical depression, sedation, and impairment. Use of kava may cause coma.	▪ Discourage use together. ▪ Monitor pt for signs and symptoms of increased CNS depression, including sedation, dizziness, ataxia, altered mental status, and respiratory depression.

lady's slipper
lemon balm
melatonin
nettle
passion flower
sassafras
skullcap
valerian

Normal laboratory test values

Hematology

Activated partial thromboplastin time
25 to 36 seconds

Hematocrit
Men: 42% to 54%
Women: 38% to 46%

Hemoglobin, total
Men: 14 to 18 g/dl
Women: 12 to 16 g/dl

Platelet count
140,000 to 400,000/mm^3

Prothrombin time
10 to 14 seconds; INR for patients on warfarin therapy, 2 to 3 (those with pediatric heart valve, 2.5 to 3.5)

Red blood cell (RBC) count
Men: 4.5 to 6.2 million/mm^3 venous blood
Women: 4.2 to 5.4 million/mm^3 venous blood

RBC indices
MCH: 26 to 32 picograms/cell
MCHC: 32 to 36 g/dl
MCV: 84 to 99 femtoliters

Reticulocyte count
0.5% to 2% of total RBC count

White blood cell (WBC) count
4,100 to 10,900/mm^3

WBC differential, blood
Basophils: 0.3% to 2%
Eosinophils: 0.3% to 7%
Lymphocytes: 16.2% to 43%
Monocytes: 0.6% to 9.6%
Neutrophils: 47.6% to 76.8%

Blood chemistry

Alanine aminotransferase
Men: 10 to 35 units/L
Women: 9 to 24 units/L

Alkaline phosphatase
Men ≥ age 19: 98 to 251 units/L
Women ages 24 to 65: 81 to 282 units/L
Women ≥ age 65: 119 to 309 units/L

Amylase
Age ≥ 18: 35 to 115 units/L

Arterial blood gases
HCO_3^-: 22 to 26 mEq/L
Pao_2: 75 to 100 mm Hg
Pao_2: 35 to 45 mm Hg
pH: 7.35 to 7.45
SaO_2: 94% to 100%

Aspartate aminotransferase
Men: 8 to 20 units/L
Women: 5 to 40 units/L

Bilirubin
Adults: direct, < 0.5 mg/dl; indirect, 1.1 mg/dl

BUN
8 to 20 mg/dl

Calcium
Men ≥ age 22, women ≥ age 19: 8.9 to 10.1 mg/dl

Carbon dioxide, total, blood
22 to 34 mEq/L

Chloride
100 to 108 mEq/L

Creatine kinase (CK)
CK-BB: None
CK-MB: 0 to 7 units/L
CK-MM: 5 to 70 units/L
Total: Men ≥ age 18, 52 to 336 units/L; women ≥ age 18, 38 to 176 units/L

Creatine
Men: 0.2 to 0.6 mg/dl
Women: 0.6 to 1 mg/dl

Creatinine
Men: 0.8 to 1.2 mg/dl
Women: 0.6 to 0.9 mg/dl

Glucose, fasting, plasma
70 to 100 mg/dl

Lactate dehydrogenase (LDH)
Total: 48 to 115 IU/L
LDH_1: 14% to 26%
LDH_2: 29% to 39%
LDH_3: 20% to 26%
LDH_4: 8% to 16%
LDH_5: 6% to 16%

Magnesium
1.5 to 2.5 mEq/L
Atomic absorption: 1.7 to 2.1 mg/dl

Phosphates
1.8 to 2.6 mEq/L
Atomic absorption: 2.5 to 4.5 mg/dl

Potassium
3.8 to 5.5 mEq/L

Protein, total
26.6 to 7.9 g/dl
Albumin fraction: 3.3 to 4.5 g/dl

Sodium
135 to 145 mEq/L

Uric acid
Men: 4.3 to 8 mg/dl
Women: 2.3 to 6 mg/dl

Unsafe herbs

The following herbs have been declared unsafe by the U.S. Food and Drug Administration (FDA) because the plants have poisonous components.

Common name	Botanical name
arnica	*Arnica montana*
belladonna	*Atropa belladonna*
bittersweet	*Solanum dulcamara*
bloodroot	*Sanguinaria canadensis*
broom-tops	*Cytisus scoparius*
buckeye	*Aesculus hippocastanum*
heliotrope	*Heliotropium europaeum*
hemlock	*Conium maculatum*
henbane	*Hyoscyamus niger*
jimsonweed	*Datura stramonium*
lily of the valley	*Convallaria majalis*
lobelia	*Lobelia inflata*
mandrake	*Mandragora officinarum*
mayapple	*Podophyllum peltatum*
mistletoe	*Phoradendron flavescens*
periwinkle	*Vinca major* and *minor*
snakeroot	*Eupatorium rugosum*
tonka bean	*Dipteryx odorata* and *coumarouna odorata*
wahoo bark	*Euonymus atropurpureus*
wormwood	*Artemisia absinthium*
yohimbe	*Corynanthe yohimbe*

Index

B

C

H

N

O

P

Q

R

S

U

V

W